Forensic Medicine: A Formula Handbook

N.B. Singh

DEDICATION

To Nature,

I dedicate this book to you, the source of all life. You are my inspiration, my teacher, and my friend.

Thank you for teaching me about the beauty of the world around me. Thank you for showing me the power of the natural world. Thank you for giving me a sense of peace and tranquillity.

I promise to do my part to protect you and your many wonders. I will teach my children about the importance of conservation and sustainability. I will work to make the world a better place for all living things.

Thank you for everything, Nature.

With love,

N.B Singh

Contents

1   Introduction   **1**

   1.1   Overview of Forensic Medicine   1

   1.2   Historical Development   1

   1.3   Scope and Importance   2

   1.4   Ethics in Forensic Medicine   3

   1.5   Legal Aspects   3

2   Forensic Autopsy   **5**

   2.1   External Examination   6

   2.2   Internal Examination   6

   2.3   Postmortem Changes   7

   2.4   Identification Techniques   8

   2.5   Time Since Death Estimation   9

   2.6   Toxicological Analysis   10

   2.7   Special Cases   11

3   Forensic Anthropology   **13**

   3.1   Bone Identification   13

   3.2   Age Estimation   14

   3.3   Sex Determination   15

   3.4   Stature Estimation   16

   3.5   Trauma Analysis   17

   3.6   Dental Identification   18

   3.7   Forensic Archaeology   19

 3.8 Mass Disasters 20

4 Forensic Odontology 21

 4.1 Dental Anatomy 21

 4.2 Bite Mark Analysis 22

 4.3 Dental Records and Identification 23

 4.4 Age Estimation from Teeth 24

 4.5 Dental Evidence in Abuse Cases 25

 4.6 Forensic Photography 26

 4.7 Digital Imaging in Forensics 27

 4.8 Legal Issues in Forensic Odontology 27

5 Forensic Pathology 29

 5.1 Overview 29

 5.2 Mechanism of Death 30

 5.3 Wound Analysis 31

 5.4 Asphyxia and Strangulation 32

 5.5 Blunt Force Injuries 33

 5.6 Sharp Force Injuries 34

 5.7 Gunshot Wounds 35

 5.8 Forensic Entomology 35

6 Forensic Toxicology 37

 6.1 Introduction to Toxicology 37

 6.2 Classes of Poisons 38

 6.3 Methods of Toxicological Analysis 39

 6.4 Drug Metabolism 40

 6.5 Toxicological Interpretation 41

 6.6 Case Studies 42

 6.7 Forensic Pharmacology 43

7 Forensic Serology and DNA Analysis 45

 7.1 Blood and Bloodstains 45

 7.2 Blood Group Systems 46

7.3   DNA Structure and Function 47

7.4   Forensic DNA Typing 48

7.5   DNA Profiling Techniques 49

7.6   Mitochondrial DNA Analysis 50

7.7   Challenges in DNA Analysis 51

8   Forensic Psychiatry   **53**

8.1   Introduction to Forensic Psychiatry 53

8.2   Criminal Responsibility 54

8.3   Competency to Stand Trial 55

8.4   Insanity Defense 56

8.5   Psychological Autopsy 57

8.6   Risk Assessment 58

8.7   Mental Health Laws 59

8.8   Psychological Profiling 60

9   Forensic Entomology   **61**

9.1   Introduction to Forensic Entomology 61

9.2   Insect Succession on Carrion 62

9.3   Role of Insects in Death Investigation 63

9.4   Forensic Arachnology 64

9.5   Applications in Legal Cases 65

9.6   Collection and Preservation of Entomological Evidence 66

9.7   Entomotoxicology 67

9.8   Forensic Acarology 68

10 Forensic Ballistics   **69**

10.1 Firearm Types and Mechanisms 70

10.2 Bullet and Cartridge Case Examination 71

10.3 Bullet Trajectory Analysis 72

10.4 Gunshot Residue Analysis 73

10.5 Firearm Identification 74

10.6 Toolmarks in Ballistics 75

10.7 Virtual Reconstruction in Ballistics 76

11 Digital Forensics   77

11.1 Introduction to Digital Forensics 77

11.2 Computer and Mobile Device Analysis 78

11.3 File Systems and Data Recovery 79

11.4 Network Forensics 80

11.5 Cybercrime Investigations 81

11.6 Forensic Analysis of Malware 82

11.7 Digital Evidence Handling 83

11.8 Legal Issues in Digital Forensics 85

12 Forensic Toxicology   87

12.1 Introduction to Toxicology 87

12.2 Classes of Poisons 88

12.3 Methods of Toxicological Analysis 89

12.4 Drug Metabolism 90

12.5 Postmortem Redistribution 91

12.6 Toxicological Interpretation 92

12.7 Case Studies 93

   12.7.1 Case 1: 93

   12.7.2 Case 2: 93

12.8 Forensic Pharmacology 94

13 Forensic Serology and DNA Analysis   95

13.1 Blood and Bloodstains 95

13.2 Blood Group Systems 96

13.3 DNA Structure and Function 97

13.4 Forensic DNA Typing 97

13.5 DNA Profiling Techniques 98

13.6 Mitochondrial DNA Analysis 99

13.7 Challenges in DNA Analysis 100

13.8 Cold Cases and DNA 100

CONTENTS

14 Forensic Anthropology   **103**

    14.1 Bone Identification 103

    14.2 Age Estimation 104

    14.3 Sex Determination 104

    14.4 Stature Estimation 105

    14.5 Trauma Analysis 106

    14.6 Dental Identification 106

    14.7 Forensic Archaeology 107

    14.8 Mass Disasters 108

15 Forensic Odontology   **109**

    15.1 Dental Anatomy 109

    15.2 Bite Mark Analysis 110

    15.3 Dental Records and Identification 110

    15.4 Age Estimation from Teeth 111

    15.5 Dental Evidence in Abuse Cases 112

    15.6 Forensic Photography 113

    15.7 Digital Imaging in Forensics 114

    15.8 Legal Issues in Forensic Odontology 115

16 Forensic Pathology   **117**

    16.1 Overview 117

    16.2 Mechanism of Death 118

    16.3 Wound Analysis 119

    16.4 Asphyxia and Strangulation 119

    16.5 Blunt Force Injuries 120

    16.6 Sharp Force Injuries 121

    16.7 Gunshot Wounds 122

    16.8 Forensic Entomology 122

17 Forensic Toxicology   **125**

    17.1 Introduction to Toxicology 125

    17.2 Classes of Poisons 126

17.3 Methods of Toxicological Analysis 126

17.4 Drug Metabolism 127

17.5 Postmortem Redistribution 128

17.6 Toxicological Interpretation 129

17.7 Case Studies 130

17.8 Forensic Pharmacology 130

18 Forensic Serology and DNA Analysis   **133**

18.1 Blood and Bloodstains 133

18.2 Blood Group Systems 134

18.3 DNA Structure and Function 135

18.4 Forensic DNA Typing 136

18.5 DNA Profiling Techniques 137

18.6 Mitochondrial DNA Analysis 138

18.7 Challenges in DNA Analysis 139

18.8 Cold Cases and DNA 140

19 Forensic Psychiatry   **141**

19.1 Introduction to Forensic Psychiatry 141

19.2 Criminal Responsibility 142

19.3 Competency to Stand Trial 142

19.4 Insanity Defense 143

19.5 Psychological Autopsy 144

19.6 Risk Assessment 144

19.7 Mental Health Laws 145

19.8 Psychological Profiling 146

20 Forensic Ballistics   **147**

20.1 Introduction to Forensic Ballistics 147

20.2 Firearm Types and Mechanisms 148

20.3 Bullet and Cartridge Case Examination 148

20.4 Bullet Trajectory Analysis 149

20.5 Gunshot Residue Analysis 150

20.6 Firearm Identification 150

20.7 Toolmarks in Ballistics 151

20.8 Virtual Reconstruction in Ballistics 152

21 Digital Forensics   155

21.1 Introduction to Digital Forensics 155

21.2 Computer and Mobile Device Analysis 156

21.3 File Systems and Data Recovery 156

21.4 Network Forensics 157

21.5 Cybercrime Investigations 158

21.6 Forensic Analysis of Malware 159

21.7 Digital Evidence Handling 160

21.8 Legal Issues in Digital Forensics 160

22 Conclusion   163

22.1 Summary of Key Findings 163

22.2 Contributions to Forensic Medicine 164

22.3 Challenges and Future Directions 164

22.4 Closing Remarks 165

PREFACE

Welcome to "Forensic Medicine: A Formula Handbook." This handbook is designed to serve as a comprehensive and accessible guide to the essential formulas, principles, and concepts in the field of forensic medicine. Whether you are a seasoned forensic professional, a student, or someone with a keen interest in the intersection of medicine and the law, this handbook aims to provide you with a valuable resource for quick reference and understanding.

Purpose of the Handbook

Forensic medicine is a dynamic and multidisciplinary field that requires a deep understanding of medical, legal, and investigative principles. In the pursuit of justice, forensic professionals often encounter complex scenarios that demand precise calculations, analyses, and interpretations. This handbook is crafted with the purpose of condensing crucial forensic information into concise and easy-to-understand formulas, allowing practitioners to navigate the intricacies of their work with efficiency.

Key Features

- **Comprehensive Coverage:** The handbook covers a wide array of forensic disciplines, including forensic toxicology, serology, DNA analysis, anthropology, psychiatry, ballistics, and more. Each section presents key formulas and concepts relevant to the respective field.

- **Quick Reference:** Formulas are presented in a clear and organized manner, facilitating rapid reference during investigations, research, or educational pursuits.

- **Accessible Language:** The content is written in a language that balances technical accuracy with accessibility, ensuring that both seasoned professionals and newcomers to the field can benefit from the handbook.

- **LaTeX Format:** The use of LaTeX allows for easy customization, enabling users to adapt and expand the handbook according to their specific needs.

How to Use This Handbook

Each chapter is dedicated to a specific subfield within forensic medicine. Formulas are presented using LaTeX, allowing for seamless integration into documents and presentations. Feel free to explore, adapt, and build upon the content provided here. This handbook is a living document, and your feedback and contributions are highly encouraged.

Thank you for choosing "Forensic Medicine: A Formula Handbook." May this resource empower you in your pursuit of truth, justice, and excellence in forensic medicine.

Chapter 1

Introduction

1.1 Overview of Forensic Medicine

Forensic Medicine involves the application of medical knowledge to legal issues. It encompasses various formulas and techniques to investigate and analyze evidence.

Key Concepts:

- PMI = Time of Death - Postmortem Interval estimation.

- DNA Analysis + Serology = Identification - Utilizing genetic information.

- Toxicology + Pathology = Cause of Death - Identifying poisonous substances.

Chemical Equations:

- Bloodstain Analysis: $Hb + O_2 \longrightarrow HbO_2$ - Hemoglobin and oxygen interaction.

- Toxicology Reaction: $X + Y \longrightarrow Z$ - Generic representation of toxic reactions.

Understanding these formulas is crucial for forensic professionals in solving legal cases.

1.2 Historical Development

The field of Forensic Medicine has evolved through key historical milestones. One can grasp its development through fundamental formulas and concepts:

- **Medico-Legal Death Investigation:**

$$\text{Medico-Legal Death} = \text{Medical Findings} + \text{Legal Investigation}$$

- **Birth of Forensic Toxicology:**

$$\text{Toxicology} = \text{Poison Identification} + \text{Dose-Response Relationships}$$

- **Introduction of Fingerprints:**

$$\text{Fingerprint Individuality} = \text{Ridge Patterns} + \text{Minutiae Points}$$

- **DNA Revolution:**

$$\text{DNA Profiling} = \text{PCR Amplification} + \text{Gel Electrophoresis}$$

Understanding these historical foundations provides insight into the interdisciplinary nature of forensic medicine.

1.3   Scope and Importance

Forensic Medicine encompasses a vast scope and holds significant importance in legal and medical domains. Let's capture its essence through essential formulas and concepts:

- **Scope of Forensic Medicine:**

$$\text{Scope} = \text{Medicine} + \text{Law} + \text{Science} + \text{Technology}$$

- **Importance of Time Since Death Estimation:**

$$\text{Time Since Death} = \text{Postmortem Changes} + \text{Environmental Factors}$$

- **Forensic Toxicology in Legal Investigations:**

$$\text{Legal Implications} = \text{Toxicology Reports} + \text{Expert Testimonies}$$

- **Role of Forensic Anthropology in Identification:**

$$\text{Identification} = \text{Anthropological Parameters} + \text{Biological Profiles}$$

Understanding the scope and importance of forensic medicine requires a holistic approach, integrating medicine, law, and scientific methodologies.

1.4   Ethics in Forensic Medicine

Ethics plays a crucial role in guiding the principles of Forensic Medicine. Let's distill its essence through essential formulas and concepts:

- **Principles of Medical Ethics:**

$$\text{Medical Ethics} = \text{Autonomy} + \text{Beneficence} + \text{Non-Maleficence} + \text{Justice}$$

- **Forensic Autopsy Ethics:**

$$\text{Autopsy Ethics} = \text{Respect for the Deceased} + \text{Family Consent} + \text{Thorough Examination}$$

- **Ethical Handling of Evidence:**

$$\text{Evidence Integrity} = \text{Chain of Custody} + \text{No Tampering} + \text{Unbiased Reporting}$$

- **Privacy and Confidentiality in Forensic Psychiatry:**

$$\text{Confidentiality} = \text{Patient Privacy} + \text{Legal Exceptions}$$

Adhering to ethical principles ensures the integrity and credibility of forensic practices, fostering trust within the legal and medical communities.

1.5   Legal Aspects

The legal aspects of forensic medicine involve key principles and considerations. Let's express them through simplified formulas and concepts:

- **Legal Responsibility:**

$$\text{Legal Responsibility} = \text{Ethical Standards} + \text{Professional Conduct}$$

- **Chain of Custody in Evidence Handling:**

$$\text{Chain of Custody} = \text{Collection Procedures} + \text{Documentation}$$

- **Expert Witness Testimony:**

$$\text{Credibility of Testimony} = \text{Qualifications} + \text{Impartiality}$$

- **Admissibility of Evidence:**

$$\text{Legal Acceptance} = \text{Relevance} + \text{Reliability}$$

Understanding the legal aspects is crucial for forensic practitioners to maintain integrity and contribute effectively to legal proceedings.

Chapter 2

Forensic Autopsy

- **External Examination:**

$$\text{External Examination} = \text{Visual Inspection} + \text{Measurements}$$

- **Internal Examination:**

$$\text{Internal Examination} = \text{Organ Inspection} + \text{Tissue Sampling}$$

- **Postmortem Changes Analysis:**

$$\text{Postmortem Changes} = \text{Temperature} + \text{Decomposition Rate}$$

- **Identification Techniques:**

$$\text{Identification} = \text{Fingerprints} + \text{Dental Records}$$

- **Time Since Death Estimation:**

$$\text{Time Since Death} = \text{Algor Mortis} + \text{Rigor Mortis}$$

- **Toxicological Analysis:**

$$\text{Toxicological Analysis} = \text{Blood Samples} + \text{Chemical Analysis}$$

- **Special Cases Consideration:**

$$\text{Special Cases} = \text{Infants} + \text{Trauma Victims}$$

Mastering the basic procedures is fundamental for accurate forensic autopsy examinations.

2.1   External Examination

The external examination in forensic autopsies involves critical observations and measurements. Let's simplify this process using essential formulas and concepts:

- **Visual Inspection:**

$$\text{Visual Inspection} = \text{Color} + \text{Bruises} + \text{Wounds}$$

- **Measurements:**

$$\text{Measurements} = \text{Body Length} + \text{Body Weight} + \text{Head Circumference}$$

- **Identification Signs:**

$$\text{Identification Signs} = \text{Scars} + \text{Tattoos} + \text{Unique Features}$$

- **Clothing Examination:**

$$\text{Clothing Examination} = \text{Blood Stains} + \text{Fiber Analysis}$$

- **External Injuries Analysis:**

$$\text{External Injuries} = \text{Contusions} + \text{Abrasions} + \text{Lacerations}$$

- **Signs of Decomposition:**

$$\text{Decomposition Signs} = \text{Odor} + \text{Insect Activity} + \text{Skin Changes}$$

Meticulous external examination is crucial for initial insights into the cause and circumstances of death.

2.2   Internal Examination

The internal examination in forensic autopsies involves detailed scrutiny of internal organs. Let's simplify this process using essential formulas and concepts:

- **Organ Inspection:**

$$\text{Organ Inspection} = \text{Heart} + \text{Lungs} + \text{Liver} + \text{Kidneys}$$

- **Tissue Sampling:**

$$\text{Tissue Sampling} = \text{Biopsy} + \text{Microscopic Examination}$$

- **Fluid Analysis:**

$$\text{Fluid Analysis} = \text{Cerebrospinal Fluid} + \text{Pleural Fluid} + \text{Peritoneal Fluid}$$

- **Vascular Examination:**

$$\text{Vascular Examination} = \text{Blood Vessels} + \text{Aneurysms} + \text{Thrombosis}$$

- **Cavity Exploration:**

$$\text{Cavity Exploration} = \text{Thoracic Cavity} + \text{Abdominal Cavity} + \text{Cranial Cavity}$$

- **Bone Marrow Examination:**

$$\text{Bone Marrow Examination} = \text{Biopsy} + \text{Hematological Analysis}$$

- **Toxicological Analysis:**

$$\text{Toxicological Analysis} = \text{Organ Samples} + \text{Chemical Analysis}$$

Thorough internal examination provides crucial insights into the physiological state and potential causes of death.

2.3 Postmortem Changes

Understanding postmortem changes is essential in forensic autopsies. Let's simplify this topic using essential formulas and concepts:

- **Algor Mortis (Body Cooling):**

$$\text{Algor Mortis} = \text{Initial Body Temperature} - \text{Room Temperature}$$

- **Rigor Mortis (Muscle Stiffening):**

$$\text{Rigor Mortis} = \text{Formation of Cross-Bridges in Muscle Fibers}$$

- **Livor Mortis (Lividity):**

$$\text{Livor Mortis} = \text{Blood Pooling in Dependent Areas} + \text{Gravity}$$

- **Postmortem Decomposition:**

$$\text{Decomposition} = \text{Autolysis} + \text{Putrefaction}$$

- **Insect Activity:**

$$\text{Insect Activity} = \text{Blow Fly Life Cycle} + \text{Maggot Development}$$

- **Adipocere Formation:**

$$\text{Adipocere Formation} = \text{Hydrolysis of Fats} + \text{Microbial Activity}$$

- **Mummification:**

$$\text{Mummification} = \text{Desiccation} + \text{Preservation}$$

Understanding these changes aids in estimating the postmortem interval and circumstances surrounding the death.

2.4 Identification Techniques

Effective identification techniques are crucial in forensic autopsies. Let's simplify this topic using essential formulas and concepts:

- **Fingerprint Identification:**

$$\text{Fingerprint Identification} = \text{Unique Ridge Patterns} + \text{Minutiae Points}$$

- **Dental Records Matching:**

$$\text{Dental Records Matching} = \text{Dental Formulas} + \text{Tooth Morphology}$$

- **DNA Profiling:**

$$\text{DNA Profiling} = \text{PCR Amplification} + \text{Gel Electrophoresis}$$

- **Facial Recognition:**

$$\text{Facial Recognition} = \text{Biometric Measurements} + \text{Computer Algorithms}$$

- **Tattoo and Scar Analysis:**

$$\text{Tattoo and Scar Analysis} = \text{Pattern Recognition} + \text{Location Identification}$$

- **Personal Items Examination:**

$$\text{Personal Items Examination} = \text{Clothing} + \text{Accessories}$$

- **Medical Implants and Prosthetics:**

$$\text{Identification through Implants} = \text{Serial Numbers} + \text{Manufacturer Records}$$

Utilizing these identification techniques aids in establishing the identity of the deceased in forensic investigations.

2.5 Time Since Death Estimation

Estimating the time since death is a critical aspect of forensic autopsies. Let's simplify this topic using essential formulas and concepts:

- **Algor Mortis (Body Cooling):**

$$\text{Algor Mortis} = \text{Initial Body Temperature} - \text{Room Temperature}$$

- **Rigor Mortis (Muscle Stiffening):**

$$\text{Rigor Mortis} = \text{Formation of Cross-Bridges in Muscle Fibers}$$

- **Livor Mortis (Lividity):**

$$\text{Livor Mortis} = \text{Blood Pooling in Dependent Areas} + \text{Gravity}$$

- **Insect Succession:**

$$\text{Insect Succession} = \text{Time-Dependent Insect Colonization} + \text{Species Identification}$$

- **DNA Degradation:**

$$\text{DNA Degradation} = \text{Postmortem Interval} + \text{Temperature Factors}$$

- **Forensic Entomology:**

$$\text{Time Since Death} = \text{Insect Development Stages} + \text{Environmental Conditions}$$

- **Body Decomposition Rates:**

$$\text{Decomposition Rates} = \text{Temperature} + \text{Humidity} + \text{Soil Characteristics}$$

Utilizing these methods aids in approximating the time elapsed since the occurrence of death in forensic investigations.

2.6   Toxicological Analysis

Toxicological analysis plays a crucial role in forensic autopsies. Let's simplify this topic using essential formulas and concepts:

- **Blood-Alcohol Concentration (BAC):**

$$\text{BAC} = \frac{\text{Alcohol in Blood}}{Blood Volume} \times 100$$

- **Drug Metabolism:**

$$\text{Drug Metabolism} = \text{Liver Enzymes} + \text{Metabolites Formation}$$

- **Toxicity Assessment:**

$$\text{Toxicity} = \text{Dose} \nabla \cdot \text{Body Weight}$$

- **Poisoning Analysis:**

$$\text{Poisoning Analysis} = \text{Symptoms} + \text{Toxic Agent Identification}$$

- **Gas Chromatography-Mass Spectrometry (GC-MS):**

$$\text{GC-MS Analysis} = \text{Sample Vaporization} + \text{Separation in GC} + \text{Mass Spectrometry}$$

- **Immunoassay Techniques:**

$$\text{Immunoassay Techniques} = \text{Antigen-Antibody Interactions} + \text{Colorimetric Detection}$$

- **Toxicological Interpretation:**

$$\text{Toxicological Interpretation} = \text{Clinical Symptoms} + \text{Laboratory Findings}$$

Utilizing these methods aids in identifying and quantifying toxic substances in the body during forensic examinations.

2.7 Special Cases

Handling special cases in forensic autopsies requires unique considerations. Let's simplify this topic using essential formulas and concepts:

- **Infants and Neonates:**

$$\text{Infant Age Estimation} = \text{Developmental Milestones} + \text{Skeletal Growth}$$

- **Trauma Victims:**

$$\text{Trauma Severity} = \text{Force Applied} \nabla \cdot \text{Surface Area}$$

- **Burn Victims:**

$$\text{Burn Depth Assessment} = \text{Degree of Tissue Damage} + \text{Surface Area}$$

- **Water-Related Deaths:**

$$\text{Drowning Analysis} = \text{Water Aspiration} + \text{Postmortem Water Absorption}$$

- **Electrocution Cases:**

$$\text{Electrocution Analysis} = \text{Voltage} \times \text{Current} \times \text{Duration}$$

- **Drug Overdoses:**

$$\text{Toxicological Analysis} = \text{Drug Levels in Blood} + \text{Metabolism Rates}$$

- **Homicide Cases:**

$$\text{Crime Scene Reconstruction} = \text{Blood Spatter Patterns} + \text{Weapon Analysis}$$

Understanding and applying these methods are crucial in addressing the complexities of special cases in forensic autopsies.

Chapter 3

Forensic Anthropology

3.1   Bone Identification

Bone identification is a fundamental aspect of forensic anthropology. Let's simplify this topic using essential formulas and concepts:

- **Bone Density Analysis:**
$$\text{Bone Density} = \frac{\text{Bone Mass}}{\text{Bone Volume}}$$

- **Osteometry for Age Estimation:**
$$\text{Estimated Age} = \text{Bone Length} + \text{Cranial Suture Closure}$$

- **Sex Determination from Pelvic Bones:**
$$\text{Sex Determination} = \text{Pelvic Width} + \text{Sacrum Characteristics}$$

- **Stature Estimation from Long Bones:**
$$\text{Stature Estimation} = \text{Long Bone Length} + \text{Regression Formulas}$$

- **Dental Morphology:**
$$\text{Dental Morphology} = \text{Cusp Patterns} + \text{Tooth Shape}$$

- **Trauma Analysis:**

$$\text{Trauma Analysis} = \text{Fracture Patterns} + \text{Blunt Force Trauma}$$

- **Determination of Ancestry:**

$$\text{Ancestry Determination} = \text{Skull Morphology} + \text{Facial Features}$$

Mastering bone identification techniques is essential for reconstructing biological profiles in forensic anthropology.

3.2   Age Estimation

Age estimation is a critical aspect of forensic anthropology. Let's simplify this topic using essential formulas and concepts:

- **Epiphyseal Union in Long Bones:**

$$\text{Age} = \text{Epiphyseal Union} + \text{Bone Length}$$

- **Cranial Suture Closure:**

$$\text{Age} = \text{Suture Closure} + \text{Skull Morphology}$$

- **Dental Development:**

$$\text{Age} = \text{Tooth Eruption Patterns} + \text{Root Formation}$$

- **Pubic Symphysis Changes:**

$$\text{Age} = \text{Symphyseal Surface Changes} + \text{Pelvic Morphology}$$

- **Auricular Surface Aging:**

$$\text{Age} = \text{Auricular Surface Changes} + \text{Iliac Crest Morphology}$$

- **Cervical Vertebrae Changes:**

$$\text{Age} = \text{Cervical Vertebrae Fusion} + \text{Vertebral Morphology}$$

- **Osteon Count in Long Bones:**

$$\text{Age} = \text{Osteon Count} + \text{Bone Microstructure}$$

Utilizing these age estimation techniques aids in constructing accurate biological profiles in forensic anthropology.

3.3 Sex Determination

Sex determination is a key aspect of forensic anthropology. Let's simplify this topic using essential formulas and concepts:

- **Pelvic Morphology:**

$$\text{Sex} = \text{Pelvic Width} + \text{Sacrum Characteristics}$$

- **Cranial Features:**

$$\text{Sex} = \text{Skull Morphology} + \text{Mandibular Structure}$$

- **Morphometric Analysis:**

$$\text{Sex} = \text{Biometric Measurements} + \text{Statistical Analysis}$$

- **Dental Characteristics:**

$$\text{Sex} = \text{Cusp Patterns} + \text{Tooth Size}$$

- **Postcranial Skeleton Analysis:**

$$\text{Sex} = \text{Long Bone Dimensions} + \text{Epiphyseal Union}$$

- **Genetic Markers Identification:**

$$\text{Sex} = \text{DNA Analysis} + \text{Presence of Sex Chromosomes}$$

- **Anthroposcopic Analysis:**

$$\text{Sex} = \text{External Genitalia Inspection} + \text{Secondary Sexual Characteristics}$$

Utilizing these sex determination techniques aids in constructing accurate biological profiles in forensic anthropology.

3.4 Stature Estimation

Estimating stature is a crucial aspect of forensic anthropology. Let's simplify this topic using essential formulas and concepts:

- **Long Bone Lengths:**

$$\text{Stature} = \text{Femur Length} + \text{Tibia Length} + \text{Humerus Length}$$

- **Regression Formulas:**

$$\text{Stature} = a + (b \times \text{Long Bone Length})$$

- **Proportional Indices:**

$$\text{Stature Index} = \frac{\text{Long Bone Length}}{\text{Stature}}$$

- **Differential Lengths:**

$$\text{Stature} = \text{Average Long Bone Length} \times \text{Multiplier}$$

- **Photogrammetric Techniques:**

$$\text{Stature} = \text{Photogrammetric Measurements} + \text{Scale Factors}$$

- **Applicability of Population-Specific Formulas:**

$$\text{Stature Estimation} = \text{Population-Specific Regression Equations} + \text{Demographic Considerations}$$

- **Principal Component Analysis (PCA):**

$$\text{Stature} = \text{Principal Components} + \text{Factor Loadings}$$

Utilizing these stature estimation techniques aids in reconstructing the physical profile of individuals in forensic anthropology.

3.5 Trauma Analysis

Analyzing trauma is a critical aspect of forensic anthropology. Let's simplify this topic using essential formulas and concepts:

- **Fracture Patterns:**

$$\text{Fracture Analysis} = \text{Bone Structure} + \text{Force Applied}$$

- **Blunt Force Trauma:**

$$\text{Blunt Force Trauma} = \text{Contusion Patterns} + \text{Impact Analysis}$$

- **Sharp Force Trauma:**

$$\text{Sharp Force Trauma} = \text{Incision Patterns} + \text{Tool Mark Analysis}$$

- **Gunshot Trauma:**

$$\text{Gunshot Trauma} = \text{Bullet Velocity} + \text{Tissue Penetration Depth}$$

- **Craniometric Analysis:**

$$\text{Craniometric Measurements} = \text{Cranial Fracture Analysis} + \text{Impact Force}$$

- **Projectile Trauma:**

$$\text{Projectile Trauma} = \text{Trajectory Analysis} + \text{Wound Morphology}$$

- **Biomechanical Analysis:**

$$\text{Biomechanical Analysis} = \text{Stress Distribution} + \text{Bone Strength}$$

Utilizing these trauma analysis techniques aids in reconstructing events and understanding the impact on skeletal remains in forensic anthropology.

3.6 Dental Identification

Dental identification is a vital aspect of forensic anthropology. Let's simplify this topic using essential formulas and concepts:

- **Dental Morphology:**

$$\text{Dental Morphology} = \text{Cusp Patterns} + \text{Tooth Shape}$$

- **Dental Formulas:**

$$\text{Dental Formulas} = \text{Incisors} + \text{Canines} + \text{Premolars} + \text{Molars}$$

- **Tooth Eruption Patterns:**

$$\text{Tooth Eruption Patterns} = \text{Chronology} + \text{Sequential Emergence}$$

- **Dental Records Matching:**

$$\text{Dental Records Matching} = \text{Tooth Numbers} + \text{Filling Patterns}$$

- **Antemortem vs. Postmortem Comparisons:**

$$\text{Comparative Analysis} = \text{Antemortem Records} + \text{Postmortem Examination}$$

- **Radiographic Analysis:**

$$\text{Radiographic Comparisons} = \text{X-ray Images} + \text{Odontometrics}$$

- **Dental Impressions:**

$$\text{Dental Impressions} = \text{Bite Marks} + \text{Dental Arch Reconstruction}$$

Leveraging these dental identification techniques is crucial for establishing the identity of individuals in forensic anthropology.

3.7 Forensic Archaeology

Forensic archaeology is a critical aspect of forensic anthropology. Let's simplify this topic using essential formulas and concepts:

- **Stratigraphy Analysis:**

$$\text{Stratigraphy Analysis} = \text{Layered Deposits} + \text{Chronological Sequence}$$

- **Site Mapping:**

$$\text{Site Mapping} = \text{Grid System} + \text{Three-Dimensional Coordinates}$$

- **Taphonomy Principles:**

$$\text{Taphonomy} = \text{Postmortem Processes} + \text{Environmental Interactions}$$

- **Excavation Techniques:**

$$\text{Excavation Techniques} = \text{Grid Troweling} + \text{Feature Documentation}$$

- **Artifact Analysis:**

$$\text{Artifact Analysis} = \text{Cultural Material Identification} + \text{Contextual Significance}$$

- **Ground-Penetrating Radar (GPR):**

$$\text{GPR Survey} = \text{Electromagnetic Waves} + \text{Subsurface Feature Detection}$$

- **Faunal Analysis:**

$$\text{Faunal Analysis} = \text{Animal Remains} + \text{Cultural and Ecological Context}$$

Understanding these forensic archaeology techniques is crucial for recovering, analyzing, and interpreting evidence in anthropological investigations.

3.8   Mass Disasters

Dealing with mass disasters is a challenging aspect of forensic anthropology. Let's simplify this topic using essential formulas and concepts:

- **Victim Enumeration:**

$$\text{Victim Enumeration} = \text{Population Density} \times \text{Affected Area}$$

- **Mortuary Services Coordination:**

$$\text{Mortuary Services} = \text{Body Reception} + \text{Identification Process}$$

- **Data Management:**

$$\text{Data Management} = \text{Digital Records} + \text{Biometric Identifiers}$$

- **DNA Profiling:**

$$\text{DNA Profiling} = \text{High-Throughput Sequencing} + \text{Comparative Analysis}$$

- **Ante Mortem Records Compilation:**

$$\text{Ante Mortem Records} = \text{Medical Records} + \text{Photographs} + \text{Dental Records}$$

- **Temporary Morgue Setup:**

$$\text{Temporary Morgue} = \text{Body Preservation} + \text{Forensic Pathologists}$$

- **Public Health Measures:**

$$\text{Public Health Measures} = \text{Disease Control} + \text{Decontamination Protocols}$$

Effectively managing mass disasters involves a multidisciplinary approach, including advanced data techniques and rapid identification processes.

Chapter 4

Forensic Odontology

4.1 Dental Anatomy

Understanding dental anatomy is crucial in forensic odontology. Let's simplify this topic using essential formulas and concepts:

- **Tooth Numbering Systems:**

$$\text{Tooth Number} = \text{Arch} + \text{Quadrant} + \text{Tooth Position}$$

- **Dental Surfaces:**

$$\text{Dental Surfaces} = \text{Occlusal} + \text{Buccal} + \text{Lingual} + \text{Mesial} + \text{Distal}$$

- **Crown and Root Structure:**

$$\text{Tooth Structure} = \text{Crown} + \text{Neck} + \text{Root}$$

- **Dental Tissues:**

$$\text{Dental Tissues} = \text{Enamel} + \text{Dentin} + \text{Pulp}$$

- **Dental Formula:**

$$\text{Dental Formula} = \text{Incisors} + \text{Canines} + \text{Premolars} + \text{Molars}$$

- **Tooth Eruption Sequence:**

$$\text{Eruption Sequence} = \text{Primary Teeth} + \text{Permanent Teeth}$$

- **Root Canal Morphology:**

$$\text{Root Canal Morphology} = \text{Number of Canals} + \text{Canal Configurations}$$

Mastery of dental anatomy is essential for accurate dental identification and analysis in forensic odontology.

4.2   Bite Mark Analysis

Bite mark analysis is a crucial aspect of forensic odontology. Let's simplify this topic using essential formulas and concepts:

- **Dental Impressions Comparison:**

$$\text{Comparison} = \text{Bite Marks} + \text{Suspect's Dental Impressions}$$

- **Individual Tooth Characteristics:**

$$\text{Identification} = \text{Tooth Width} + \text{Tooth Shape} + \text{Incisal Patterns}$$

- **Bite Mark Depth Analysis:**

$$\text{Depth Analysis} = \text{Impression Depth} + \text{Tissue Response}$$

- **Three-Dimensional Bite Mark Imaging:**

$$\text{Imaging} = \text{Photogrammetry} + \text{Digital Surface Scanning}$$

- **Comparative Dental Photographic Analysis:**

$$\text{Photographic Analysis} = \text{Bite Mark Photographs} + \text{Dental Records}$$

- **Bite Mark Classification:**

$$\text{Classification} = \text{Human vs. Animal Bites} + \text{Pattern Recognition}$$

- **Age Estimation from Bite Marks:**

$$\text{Age Estimation} = \text{Bite Mark Features} + \text{Dental Eruption Patterns}$$

Mastering bite mark analysis techniques is vital for linking bite marks to specific individuals in forensic odontology.

4.3 Dental Records and Identification

Dental records and identification are vital in forensic odontology. Let's simplify this topic using essential formulas and concepts:

- **Antemortem Dental Records Compilation:**

$$\text{Antemortem Records} = \text{Medical History} + \text{Orthodontic Records} + \text{Radiographs}$$

- **Postmortem Dental Examination:**

$$\text{Postmortem Examination} = \text{Photographic Documentation} + \text{Bite Mark Analysis} + \text{Radiographic Comparison}$$

- **Dental Charting:**

$$\text{Dental Chart} = \text{Tooth Numbering} + \text{Restorations} + \text{Missing Teeth}$$

- **Dental Radiography:**

$$\text{Radiographic Analysis} = \text{Periapical Radiographs} + \text{Bitewing Radiographs} + \text{Panoramic Radiographs}$$

- **Dental Photographs:**

$$\text{Photographic Comparison} = \text{Facial Images} + \text{Intraoral Photographs} + \text{Extraoral Photographs}$$

- **Dental Impressions and Casts:**

$$\text{Impression Analysis} = \text{Dental Impressions} + \text{Casting Techniques}$$

- **Biometric Identification:**

$$\text{Biometric Analysis} = \text{Dental Metrics} + \text{Odontometrics} + \text{Digital Imaging}$$

Effectively utilizing dental records and identification methods is essential for accurate victim identification in forensic odontology.

4.4   Age Estimation from Teeth

Estimating age from teeth is a crucial aspect of forensic odontology. Let's simplify this topic using essential formulas and concepts:

- **Tooth Eruption Sequences:**

$$\text{Eruption Sequence} = \text{Chronology of Tooth Emergence} + \text{Tooth Development}$$

- **Dental Developmental Stages:**

$$\text{Developmental Stages} = \text{Crown Formation} + \text{Root Formation} + \text{Tooth Mineralization}$$

- **Root Dentin Transparency:**

$$\text{Transparency Analysis} = \text{Root Dentin Transparency} + \text{Aging Factors}$$

- **Wear Patterns and Attrition:**

$$\text{Attrition Analysis} = \text{Wear Patterns} + \text{Tooth Surface Examination}$$

- **Cementum Annulation:**

$$\text{Cementum Analysis} = \text{Annulation Patterns} + \text{Microscopic Examination}$$

- **Dental Radiographic Analysis:**

$$\text{Radiographic Assessment} = \text{Root Development} + \text{Apical Closure}$$

- **Dental Metrics and Odontometrics:**

$$\text{Odontometric Measurements} = \text{Crown Height} + \text{Cervical Diameter} + \text{Tooth Dimensions}$$

Utilizing these age estimation techniques from teeth assists in constructing accurate biological profiles in forensic odontology.

4.5 Dental Evidence in Abuse Cases

Utilizing dental evidence in abuse cases is critical in forensic odontology. Let's simplify this topic using essential concepts:

- **Bite Mark Analysis:**

$$\text{Bite Mark Identification} = \text{Bite Mark Patterns} + \text{Comparative Analysis}$$

- **Dental Trauma Assessment:**

$$\text{Trauma Analysis} = \text{Fracture Patterns} + \text{Impact Force Assessment}$$

- **Oral Soft Tissue Injuries:**

$$\text{Soft Tissue Examination} = \text{Lacerations} + \text{Contusions} + \text{Abrasions}$$

- **Dental Radiographic Signs of Abuse:**

$$\text{Radiographic Evidence} = \text{Periapical Radiographs} + \text{Crown or Root Fractures}$$

- **Dental Age Assessment:**

$$\text{Age Estimation} = \text{Developmental Stages} + \text{Dental Metrics}$$

- **Cultural and Ethnic Considerations:**

$$\text{Cultural Sensitivity} = \text{Ethnic Dental Variations} + \text{Population-Specific Norms}$$

- **Documentation and Legal Reporting:**

$$\text{Forensic Report} = \text{Detailed Documentation} + \text{Expert Testimony}$$

Effectively utilizing dental evidence in abuse cases requires a comprehensive approach, considering both physical and radiographic findings.

4.6   Forensic Photography

Effective forensic photography is crucial in forensic odontology. Let's simplify this topic using essential concepts:

- **Scale and Reference Calibration:**

$$\text{Scale Calibration} = \frac{\text{Actual Measurement}}{\text{Photograph Measurement}}$$

- **Standardized Lighting Conditions:**

$$\text{Lighting Intensity} = \frac{\text{Light Output}}{\text{Distance}^2}$$

- **Depth of Field:**

$$\text{Depth of Field} = \frac{\text{Aperture Size} \times \text{Distance to Subject}}{\text{Focal Length}^2}$$

- **Photographic Documentation of Dental Anatomy:**

$$\text{Intraoral Photography} = \text{Proper Angulation} + \text{Focus on Dental Features}$$

- **Bite Mark Photography:**

$$\text{Bite Mark Documentation} = \text{Consistent Lighting} + \text{Macro Photography}$$

- **Close-up Photography Techniques:**

$$\text{Close-up Shots} = \text{Magnification} + \text{Clear Focal Point}$$

- **Digital Imaging Considerations:**

$$\text{Digital Forensic Imaging} = \text{Resolution} + \text{Metadata Preservation}$$

Mastering forensic photography techniques is essential for accurate documentation and analysis in forensic odontology.

4.7 Digital Imaging in Forensics

Digital imaging plays a pivotal role in forensic odontology. Let's simplify this topic using essential concepts:

- **Pixel Resolution:**

$$\text{Pixel Density} = \frac{\text{Number of Pixels}}{\text{Area}}$$

- **Color Reproduction:**

$$\text{Color Accuracy} = \text{Color Depth} + \text{Color Gamut}$$

- **Metadata Preservation:**

$$\text{Metadata Integrity} = \text{Data Embedding} + \text{Digital Watermarking}$$

- **Compression Techniques:**

$$\text{Image Compression} = \text{Lossy Compression} + \text{Lossless Compression}$$

- **Three-Dimensional Imaging:**

$$\text{3D Reconstruction} = \text{Depth Sensing} + \text{Surface Mapping}$$

- **Biometric Analysis:**

$$\text{Facial Recognition} = \text{Feature Extraction} + \text{Pattern Matching}$$

- **Forensic Comparison Software:**

$$\text{Image Analysis Tools} = \text{Edge Detection} + \text{Pattern Recognition}$$

Leveraging digital imaging tools and techniques enhances the precision and efficiency of forensic odontology investigations.

4.8 Legal Issues in Forensic Odontology

Navigating legal aspects is crucial in forensic odontology. Let's simplify this topic using essential concepts:

- **Forensic Report Accuracy:**

$$\text{Report Accuracy} = \text{Thorough Documentation} + \text{Objective Language}$$

- **Expert Witness Testimony:**

$$\text{Expert Testimony} = \text{Clear Communication} + \text{Professional Demeanor}$$

- **Ethical Considerations:**

$$\text{Ethical Practice} = \text{Confidentiality} + \text{Informed Consent}$$

- **Chain of Custody Maintenance:**

$$\text{Custody Integrity} = \text{Secure Handling} + \text{Documented Transfer}$$

- **Quality Assurance Protocols:**

$$\text{Quality Standards} = \text{Regular Audits} + \text{Continuing Education}$$

- **Case Documentation Policies:**

$$\text{Case Records} = \text{Comprehensive Information} + \text{Secure Storage}$$

- **Collaboration with Legal Authorities:**

$$\text{Legal Cooperation} = \text{Timely Response} + \text{Adherence to Procedures}$$

Adhering to legal and ethical principles ensures the credibility and reliability of forensic odontology practices.

Chapter 5

Forensic Pathology

5.1   Overview

Forensic Pathology provides insights into the cause and manner of death. Let's simplify this overview using essential concepts:

- **Cause of Death Determination:**

$$\text{Cause of Death} = \text{Pathological Findings} + \text{Medical History Analysis}$$

- **Manner of Death Classification:**

$$\text{Manner of Death} = \text{Natural} + \text{Accidental} + \text{Suicidal} + \text{Homicidal} + \text{Undetermined}$$

- **Postmortem Interval Estimation:**

$$\text{Postmortem Interval} = \text{Decomposition Stages} + \text{Environmental Factors}$$

- **Toxicological Analysis:**

$$\text{Toxicology} = \text{Blood Samples} + \text{Chemical Substance Detection}$$

- **Autopsy Techniques:**

$$\text{Autopsy Examination} = \text{External Examination} + \text{Internal Examination}$$

- **Injury Pattern Analysis:**

$$\text{Injury Assessment} = \text{Wound Characteristics} + \text{Trauma Reconstruction}$$

- **Forensic Anthropological Collaboration:**

$$\text{Skeletal Examination} = \text{Bone Analysis} + \text{Identification Techniques}$$

Understanding these fundamental aspects is key to unraveling the mysteries surrounding the deceased in forensic pathology.

5.2 Mechanism of Death

Understanding the mechanism of death involves exploring physiological processes. Let's simplify this using essential concepts:

- **Cardiopulmonary Failure:**

$$\text{Mechanism} = \text{Heart Failure} + \text{Respiratory Arrest}$$

- **Hypoxia and Cellular Dysfunction:**

$$\text{Hypoxia} = \text{Oxygen Deprivation} + \text{Cellular Energy Failure}$$

- **CNS Depression and Neurological Dysfunction:**

$$\text{Neurological Dysfunction} = \text{Central Nervous System Depression} + \text{Impaired Brain Function}$$

- **Coagulation Cascade Disruption:**

$$\text{Disseminated Intravascular Coagulation (DIC)}$$

$$= \text{Abnormal Blood Clotting} + \text{Systemic Organ Failure}$$

- **Metabolic Acidosis and Organ Failure:**

$$\text{Organ Dysfunction} = \text{Metabolic Acidosis} + \text{Multi-Organ Failure}$$

- **Toxicological Mechanisms:**

$$\text{Toxic Exposure} = \text{Chemical Interactions} + \text{Organ Toxicity}$$

- **Electrolyte Imbalance:**

$$\text{Electrolyte Disruption} = \text{Ion Concentration Changes} + \text{Cellular Dysfunction}$$

Recognizing the mechanisms underlying death is critical in forensic pathology for determining the cause and contributing factors.

5.3 Wound Analysis

Analyzing wounds is crucial in forensic pathology. Let's simplify this using essential concepts:

- **Wound Classification:**

$$\text{Wound Type} = \text{Incised} + \text{Stabbed} + \text{Gunshot} + \text{Blunt Force}$$

- **Wound Shape and Characteristics:**

$$\text{Wound Characteristics} = \text{Entry vs. Exit} + \text{Abrasion Patterns} + \text{Laceration Severity}$$

- **Firearm Ballistics:**

$$\text{Projectile Motion} = \text{Velocity} + \text{Bullet Trajectory} + \text{Tissue Penetration}$$

- **Blunt Force Trauma Analysis:**

$$\text{Impact Dynamics} = \text{Force Applied} + \text{Surface Area of Impact} + \text{Fracture Patterns}$$

- **Sharp Force Injuries:**

$$\text{Sharp Force Trauma} = \text{Depth of Penetration} + \text{Wound Shape} + \text{Weapon Identification}$$

- **Patterned Injuries:**

$$\text{Pattern Analysis} = \text{Tool Mark Identification} + \text{Imprint Examination}$$

- **Postmortem Wound Changes:**

$$\text{Decompositional Effects} = \text{Postmortem Interval} + \text{Insect Activity}$$

Comprehensive wound analysis aids in reconstructing events and determining the manner of death in forensic pathology.

5.4 Asphyxia and Strangulation

Understanding asphyxia and strangulation is vital in forensic pathology. Let's simplify this using essential concepts:

- **Asphyxia Mechanisms:**

$$\text{Asphyxiation} = \text{Oxygen Deprivation} + \text{Carbon Dioxide Accumulation}$$

- **Hanging Analysis:**

$$\text{Hanging Mechanism} = \text{Suspension Dynamics} + \text{Neck Compression} + \text{Cervical Injury Assessment}$$

- **Strangulation Patterns:**

$$\text{Manual Strangulation} = \text{Hand Placement} + \text{External Pressure} + \text{Internal Neck Injuries}$$

- **Garrote Strangulation:**

$$\text{Garrote Mechanism} = \text{Tightening Force} + \text{Strangulating Device Type}$$

- **Environmental Factors:**

$$\text{Asphyxiation Risk} = \text{Confined Spaces} + \text{Gas Concentrations}$$

- **Postmortem Changes:**

$$\text{Decomposition Effects} = \text{Autolytic Changes} + \text{Insect Activity}$$

- **Forensic Evidence Documentation:**

$$\text{Forensic Report} = \text{Injury Patterns} + \text{Toxicological Findings} + \text{Scene Analysis}$$

Comprehending the mechanisms of asphyxia and strangulation aids in accurate cause-of-death determination in forensic pathology.

5.5   Blunt Force Injuries

Analyzing blunt force injuries is crucial in forensic pathology. Let's simplify this using essential concepts:

- **Force Impact Calculation:**

$$\text{Force} = \text{Mass} \times \text{Acceleration}$$

- **Energy Transfer in Trauma:**

$$\text{Kinetic Energy} = \frac{1}{2} \times \text{Mass} \times \text{Velocity}^2$$

- **Injury Severity Assessment:**

$$\text{Injury Severity} = \text{Force Applied} + \text{Surface Area of Impact}$$

- **Fracture Mechanics:**

$$\text{Fracture Analysis} = \text{Force Distribution} + \text{Bone Density}$$

- **Acceleration-Deceleration Injuries:**

$$\text{Head Injury Mechanism} = \text{Acceleration} + \text{Deceleration} + \text{Brain Trauma}$$

- **Trauma Reconstruction:**

$$\text{Event Reconstruction} = \text{Injury Patterns} + \text{Impact Dynamics}$$

- **Postmortem Changes:**

$$\text{Decomposition Effects} = \text{Soft Tissue Breakdown} + \text{Insect Activity}$$

Understanding the physics of blunt force injuries aids in reconstructing events and determining the severity of trauma in forensic pathology.

5.6   Sharp Force Injuries

Analyzing sharp force injuries is crucial in forensic pathology. Let's simplify this using essential concepts:

- **Penetration Force Calculation:**

$$\text{Penetration Force} = \text{Force Applied} \times \text{Edge Sharpness}$$

- **Wound Shape and Depth Analysis:**

$$\text{Wound Characteristics} = \text{Blade Type} + \text{Angle of Attack} + \text{Tissue Resistance}$$

- **Identification of Weapon Characteristics:**

$$\text{Weapon Type} = \text{Wound Patterns} + \text{Microscopic Examination}$$

- **Depth of Penetration Calculation:**

$$\text{Penetration Depth} = \text{Force Applied} \times \text{Blade Geometry}$$

- **Wound Healing Patterns:**

$$\text{Healing Process} = \text{Wound Edges Alignment} + \text{Tissue Repair Mechanisms}$$

- **Fatal Injury Assessment:**

$$\text{Lethal Injury Severity} = \text{Vital Organ Involvement} + \text{Hemorrhage Level}$$

- **Postmortem Changes:**

$$\text{Decomposition Effects} = \text{Wound Breakdown} + \text{Insect Activity}$$

Understanding the dynamics of sharp force injuries is essential for weapon identification and cause-of-death determination in forensic pathology.

5.7 Gunshot Wounds

Analyzing gunshot wounds is vital in forensic pathology. Let's simplify this using essential concepts:

- **Projectile Kinetic Energy:**

$$\text{Kinetic Energy} = \frac{1}{2} \times \text{Projectile Mass} \times \text{Velocity}^2$$

- **Muzzle Velocity Calculation:**

$$\text{Muzzle Velocity} = \sqrt{\frac{\text{Kinetic Energy} \times 2}{\text{Projectile Mass}}}$$

- **Terminal Ballistics:**

$$\text{Tissue Penetration} = \text{Bullet Design} + \text{Velocity Decay}$$

- **Wound Channel Characteristics:**

$$\text{Cavitation Effect} = \text{Temporary Cavity Formation} + \text{Permanent Cavity Formation}$$

- **Gunshot Residue Analysis:**

$$\text{GSR Detection} = \text{Residue Distribution} + \text{Firearm Identification}$$

- **Close Range Firearm Examination:**

$$\text{Stippling Patterns} = \text{Burn Patterns} + \text{Shot Distance Estimation}$$

- **Projectile Trajectory Reconstruction:**

$$\text{Bullet Path} = \text{Entrance Wound Analysis} + \text{Exit Wound Analysis}$$

Understanding the ballistics and characteristics of gunshot wounds is essential for forensic pathologists in determining the cause and manner of death.

5.8 Forensic Entomology

Forensic entomology plays a crucial role in estimating postmortem interval. Let's simplify this using essential concepts:

- **Blow Fly Life Cycle:**

$$\text{Development Time} = \text{Egg Hatch} + \text{Larval Instars} + \text{Pupal Stage}$$

- **Temperature-Driven Growth:**

$$\text{Development Rate} = \text{Temperature} + \text{Base Development Threshold}$$

- **Maggot Mass Temperature Estimation:**

$$\text{Maggot Mass Temperature} = \text{Ambient Temperature} + \text{Decomposition Heat}$$

- **Succession of Insect Colonization:**

$$\text{Species Succession} = \text{First Arriving Species} + \text{Subsequent Colonizers}$$

- **Entomotoxicology:**

$$\text{Chemical Analysis} = \text{Insect Tissues} + \text{Toxicological Substances}$$

- **Geographic Location Influence:**

$$\text{Geographic Factors} = \text{Climate} + \text{Local Fauna Presence}$$

- **Entomological Evidence Documentation:**

$$\text{Forensic Report} = \text{Insect Specimens Identification} + \text{Life Stage Analysis}$$

Utilizing forensic entomology aids in precise postmortem interval estimation and provides valuable evidence in forensic pathology.

Chapter 6

Forensic Toxicology

6.1 Introduction to Toxicology

Toxicology explores the adverse effects of chemicals on living organisms. Let's simplify this using essential concepts:

- **Dose-Response Relationship:**

$$\text{Effect} = \text{Dose} \times \text{Sensitivity}$$

- **Toxicity Index Calculation:**

$$\text{Toxicity Index} = \frac{\text{Lethal Dose}}{\text{Effective Dose}}$$

- **Half-Life of Elimination:**

$$\text{Elimination Half-Life} = \frac{0.693}{\text{Elimination Rate}}$$

- **Absorption and Distribution:**

$$\text{Bioavailability} = \frac{\text{Absorbed Dose}}{\text{Administered Dose}}$$

- **Metabolism and Biotransformation:**

$$\text{Metabolic Rate} = \text{Enzyme Activity} \times \text{Substrate Concentration}$$

- **Excretion Rate Calculation:**

$$\text{Excretion Rate} = \frac{\text{Amount Excreted}}{\text{Time Interval}}$$

- **Toxicokinetics:**

$$\text{Toxicant Movement} = \text{Absorption} + \text{Distribution} + \text{Metabolism} + \text{Excretion}$$

Understanding these principles is crucial in assessing the impact of toxic substances and determining their role in forensic investigations.

6.2   Classes of Poisons

Understanding different classes of poisons is crucial in forensic toxicology. Let's simplify this using essential concepts:

- **Heavy Metals:**

$$\text{Metal Toxicity} = \text{Metal Concentration} \times \text{Exposure Duration}$$

- **Alcohol and Volatile Substances:**

$$\text{Blood Alcohol Concentration (BAC)} = \frac{\text{Alcohol Amount}}{\text{Blood Volume}}$$

- **Opioids:**

$$\text{Opioid Toxicity} = \text{Opioid Receptor Binding} + \text{Respiratory Depression}$$

- **Stimulants:**

$$\text{Stimulant Effects} = \text{Increased Heart Rate} + \text{Elevated Blood Pressure}$$

- **Depressants:**

$$\text{Central Nervous System Depression} = \text{GABA Receptor Modulation} + \text{Sedation}$$

- **Anticholinergics:**

$$\text{Anticholinergic Toxicity} = \text{Acetylcholine Blockade} + \text{Dry Mouth, Dilated Pupils}$$

- **Toxic Gases:**

$$\text{Gas Exposure Toxicity} = \text{Inhalation Concentration} \times \text{Exposure Time}$$

Recognizing the characteristics and effects of various poison classes aids in identifying toxic substances and determining their impact in forensic toxicology.

6.3   Methods of Toxicological Analysis

Analyzing toxic substances requires various methods. Let's simplify this using essential concepts:

- **Gas Chromatography (GC):**

$$\text{GC Analysis} = \text{Vaporization} + \text{Separation} + \text{Detection}$$

- **Liquid Chromatography (LC):**

$$\text{LC Analysis} = \text{Mobile Phase} + \text{Stationary Phase} + \text{Detector Response}$$

- **Mass Spectrometry (MS):**

$$\text{MS Analysis} = \text{Ionization} + \text{Mass-to-Charge Ratio Determination} + \text{Detection}$$

- **Immunoassays:**

$$\text{Immunoassay} = \text{Antibody-Antigen Reaction} + \text{Signal Detection} + \text{Quantification}$$

- **Enzyme-Linked Immunosorbent Assay (ELISA):**

$$\text{ELISA Analysis} = \text{Enzyme Reaction} + \text{Color Change} + \text{Concentration Determination}$$

- **Atomic Absorption Spectroscopy (AAS):**

$$\text{AAS Analysis} = \text{Atomization} + \text{Absorption Measurement} + \text{Concentration Determination}$$

- **Nuclear Magnetic Resonance (NMR):**

$$\text{NMR Analysis} = \text{Nuclear Spin Excitation} + \text{Signal Detection} + \text{Spectrum Interpretation}$$

Utilizing these methods facilitates the accurate identification and quantification of toxic substances in forensic toxicology.

6.4   Drug Metabolism

Understanding how the body processes drugs is crucial in forensic toxicology. Let's simplify this using essential concepts:

- **Metabolic Pathways:**

$$\text{Metabolism} = \text{Phase I Reactions} + \text{Phase II Reactions}$$

- **Phase I Reactions:**

$$\text{Oxidation} = \text{Cytochrome P450 Enzymes} + \text{NADPH}$$

$$\text{Reduction} = \text{Microsomal Enzymes} + \text{Electron Donors}$$

$$\text{Hydrolysis} = \text{Esterases} + \text{Water}$$

- **Phase II Reactions:**

$$\text{Conjugation} = \text{Glucuronidation} + \text{Sulfation} + \text{Acetylation}$$

- **Enzyme Inhibition and Induction:**

$$\text{Inhibition} = \text{Competitive Inhibition} + \text{Non-Competitive Inhibition}$$

$$\text{Induction} = \text{Enzyme Activation} + \text{Gene Expression}$$

- **Half-Life Calculation:**

$$\text{Drug Half-Life} = \frac{0.693}{\text{Elimination Rate Constant}}$$

- **First-Order Kinetics:**

$$\text{Concentration} = \text{Initial Concentration} \times e^{-kt}$$

Understanding drug metabolism aids in interpreting toxicological findings and predicting the duration of drug effects in forensic toxicology.

- **Drug Redistribution Equation:**

$$\text{Redistribution Ratio} = \frac{\text{Concentration in Peripheral Tissues}}{\text{Concentration in Central Blood}}$$

- **Factors Influencing Redistribution:**

$$\text{Blood pH} + \text{Temperature} + \text{Drug Lipophilicity} + \text{Blood-Brain Barrier Permeability}$$

- **Postmortem Interval Effects:**

$$\text{Redistribution Kinetics} = \text{Time Since Death} + \text{Body Decomposition}$$

- **Calculation of Corrected Concentrations:**

$$\text{Corrected Concentration} = \frac{\text{Measured Concentration}}{\text{Redistribution Ratio}}$$

- **Tissue-Specific Redistribution:**

$$\text{Organ Redistribution Index} = \frac{\text{Concentration in Organ}}{\text{Concentration in Central Blood}}$$

- **Evaluation of Toxicity:**

$$\text{Toxic Threshold} + \text{Corrected Concentrations} + \text{Clinical Symptoms Analysis}$$

- **Postmortem Redistribution Limitations:**

$$\text{Interpretation Caution} = \text{Multiple Sampling Sites} + \text{Consistency Checks}$$

Understanding the dynamics of postmortem redistribution is essential for accurate toxicological assessments in forensic cases.

6.5 Toxicological Interpretation

Interpreting toxicological findings involves various factors. Let's simplify this using essential concepts:

- **Threshold Concentrations:**

$$\text{Toxic Threshold} = \text{Minimum Concentration for Toxic Effects}$$

- **Lethal Dose Calculation:**

$$\text{LD50} = \text{Dose at which 50\% of Subjects Die}$$

- **Therapeutic Index:**

$$\text{Therapeutic Index} = \frac{\text{Therapeutic Dose Range}}{\text{Toxic Dose Range}}$$

- **Synergistic and Antagonistic Effects:**

$$\text{Effect of Combined Substances} = \text{Summation (Synergism)} + \text{Offset (Antagonism)}$$

- **Absorption Rate Calculation:**

$$\text{Absorption Rate} = \frac{\text{Rate of Absorption}}{\text{Dosage Form Characteristics}}$$

- **Distribution and Elimination:**

$$\text{Volume of Distribution} + \text{Half-life} = \text{Drug Clearance Rate}$$

- **Metabolism Influence on Toxicity:**

$$\text{Active Metabolite Formation} + \text{Metabolism Rate} = \text{Enhanced Toxicity}$$

Understanding these parameters aids in interpreting toxicological results and determining the significance of substance concentrations in forensic cases.

6.6   Case Studies

Learning from real-world cases enhances understanding. Let's simplify this using essential concepts:

- **Case Analysis Framework:**

$$\text{Victim Information} + \text{Scene Investigation} + \text{Toxicological Findings}$$

- **Blood-Alcohol Content (BAC) Calculations:**

$$\text{BAC} = \frac{\text{Alcohol Amount}}{\text{Blood Volume}}$$

- **Multiple Substance Interaction:**

$$\text{Combined Effect} = \text{Summation (Additivity)} + \text{Interaction (Synergism/Antagonism)}$$

- **Postmortem Redistribution Considerations:**

$$\text{Redistribution Ratio} + \text{Corrected Concentrations} + \text{Interpretation Challenges}$$

- **Unexpected Metabolism Impact:**

$$\text{Metabolite Formation} + \text{Metabolism Rate Deviation} = \text{Altered Toxicity}$$

- **Therapeutic Overdose Assessment:**

$$\text{Exceeded Therapeutic Range} + \text{Clinical Symptoms} = \text{Toxicity Confirmation}$$

- **Communication of Findings:**

$$\text{Forensic Report Clarity} + \text{Expert Testimony Preparation} = \text{Legal Impact}$$

Analyzing case studies provides valuable insights into applying forensic toxicology principles in real-life scenarios.

6.7 Forensic Pharmacology

Understanding the pharmacological aspects in forensic cases is crucial. Let's simplify this using essential concepts:

- **Drug-Receptor Interaction:**

$$\text{Effect} = \text{Drug-Receptor Binding} + \text{Signal Transduction}$$

- **Dose-Response Relationship:**

$$\text{Response} = \text{Dose} + \text{Sigmoidal Curve}$$

- **Pharmacokinetics:**

$$\text{Absorption Rate} + \text{Distribution in Tissues} + \text{Metabolism Rate} + \text{Elimination Rate}$$

- **Pharmacodynamics:**

$$\text{Effect at Target Site} = \text{Drug-Receptor Interaction} + \text{Cellular Response}$$

- **Therapeutic Window:**

$$\text{Effective Dose Range} + \text{Toxic Dose Range} = \text{Optimal Therapeutic Window}$$

- **Drug Interactions:**

$$\text{Pharmacokinetic Interactions} + \text{Pharmacodynamic Interactions} = \text{Combined Effect}$$

- **Individual Variation Considerations:**

$$\text{Genetic Factors} + \text{Health Conditions} + \text{Drug Sensitivity} = \text{Response Variability}$$

Incorporating forensic pharmacology principles enhances the understanding of drug effects and aids in toxicological assessments.

Chapter 7

Forensic Serology and DNA Analysis

7.1 Blood and Bloodstains

Understanding blood and bloodstains is essential in forensic serology. Let's simplify this using essential concepts:

- **Blood Typing:**

$$\text{Blood Type} = \text{Antigen Presence} + \text{Serum Antibody Reaction}$$

- **Presumptive Blood Tests:**

$$\text{Luminol Reaction} + \text{Kastle-Meyer Test} + \text{Hemastix Reaction}$$

- **Blood Spatter Analysis:**

$$\text{Impact Angle Calculation} + \text{Bloodstain Shape Analysis} + \text{Area of Convergence}$$

- **Hemoglobin Analysis:**

$$\text{Hemoglobin Presence} + \text{Hemoglobin Species Differentiation}$$

- **Preservation of DNA in Blood:**

$$\text{EDTA Anticoagulant} + \text{Cold Storage Conditions} + \text{DNA Stability}$$

- **Y-Chromosome Analysis for Male Identification:**

$$\text{Y-Chromosome STRs} + \text{Amelogenin Gene Analysis} + \text{Male-Specific Markers}$$

- **DNA Quantification from Bloodstains:**

$$\text{Quantitative PCR (qPCR)} + \text{DNA Concentration Determination}$$

Comprehending the characteristics and analysis methods of blood and bloodstains is fundamental for accurate forensic serology and DNA investigations.

7.2   Blood Group Systems

Understanding blood group systems is crucial in forensic serology. Let's simplify this using essential concepts:

- **ABO Blood Group System:**

$$\text{Blood Type} = \text{Presence of A and/or B Antigens}+$$

$$\text{Absence or Presence of Anti-A and/or Anti-B Antibodies}$$

- **Rh Blood Group System:**

$$\text{Rh Factor} = \text{Presence or Absence of Rh (D) Antigen}$$

- **MN Blood Group System:**

$$\text{M and N Antigen Presence} + \text{Serum Antibody Reaction}$$

- **Lewis Blood Group System:**

$$\text{Lewis Antigen Presence on RBCs} + \text{Secretor or Non-Secretor Status}$$

- **Kell Blood Group System:**

$$\text{Kell Antigen Presence} + \text{Kell Antibody Reaction}$$

- **Duffy Blood Group System:**

  Duffy Antigen Presence or Absence + Resistance or Susceptibility to Malaria

- **Diego Blood Group System:**

  Diego Antigen Presence + Diego Antibody Reaction

Comprehending the characteristics of different blood group systems is essential for accurate blood typing and forensic serology analyses.

7.3 DNA Structure and Function

Understanding DNA structure and function is fundamental in forensic DNA analysis. Let's simplify this using essential concepts:

- **DNA Double Helix:**

  DNA Structure = Double Helical Model + Base Pairing (A-T, C-G)

- **DNA Replication:**

  DNA Synthesis = Complementary Base Pairing + Enzymatic Replication

- **Transcription to RNA:**

  RNA Synthesis = DNA to RNA Template Strand + RNA Polymerase

- **Genetic Code and Codons:**

  Genetic Information = Codons (3-Nucleotide Sequences) + Amino Acid Coding

- **Translation to Proteins:**

  Protein Synthesis = mRNA to Polypeptide Chain + Ribosomes and tRNA

- **DNA Repair Mechanisms:**

  Mismatch Repair + Nucleotide Excision Repair + Base Excision Repair

- **DNA Profiling Techniques:**

    PCR (Polymerase Chain Reaction) + STR (Short Tandem Repeat) Analysis + Electrophoresis

Understanding the intricacies of DNA structure and function is crucial for accurate forensic DNA analysis and identification.

7.4 Forensic DNA Typing

Forensic DNA typing involves specific methodologies and principles. Let's simplify this using essential concepts:

- **Polymerase Chain Reaction (PCR):**

$$\text{Amplification of DNA} = \text{Denaturation} + \text{Primer Annealing} + \text{Extension}$$

- **Short Tandem Repeat (STR) Analysis:**

$$\text{STR Loci} = \text{Repeating Units} + \text{Multiplex PCR} + \text{Fluorescent Labeling}$$

- **DNA Electrophoresis:**

$$\text{Separation by Size} = \text{Agarose Gel or Capillary Electrophoresis} + \text{Migration of Fragments}$$

- **Genetic Profiling and Allele Identification:**

$$\text{Genotype Determination} = \text{Pattern Analysis} + \text{Peak Height and Area Measurement}$$

- **Mitochondrial DNA (mtDNA) Analysis:**

$$\text{mtDNA Extraction} + \text{Sequencing} + \text{Maternal Lineage Identification}$$

- **Y-Chromosome Analysis:**

$$\text{Y-STR Loci Analysis} + \text{Male Lineage Identification} + \text{Paternal Inheritance}$$

- **Statistical Analysis and Probability Calculations:**

$$\text{Random Match Probability} + \text{Likelihood Ratio} + \text{Population Databases}$$

Understanding the techniques and principles of forensic DNA typing is essential for reliable and accurate DNA profiling in criminal investigations.

7.5 DNA Profiling Techniques

DNA profiling employs specific techniques for accurate identification. Let's simplify this using essential concepts:

- **Polymerase Chain Reaction (PCR):**

$$DNA\ Amplification = Denaturation + Primer\ Annealing + Extension$$

- **Short Tandem Repeat (STR) Analysis:**

$$STR\ Loci = Repeating\ Units + Multiplex\ PCR + Fluorescent\ Labeling$$

- **Capillary Electrophoresis:**

$$DNA\ Fragment\ Separation = Capillary\ Tube + Electrokinetic\ Injection + Laser\ Detection$$

- **Single Nucleotide Polymorphism (SNP) Analysis:**

$$SNP\ Genotyping = Allele\ Discrimination + Mass\ Spectrometry\ Detection$$

- **Mitochondrial DNA (mtDNA) Sequencing:**

$$mtDNA\ Amplification + Sanger\ Sequencing + Haplogroup\ Determination$$

- **Y-Chromosome Analysis:**

$$Y\text{-}STR\ Loci\ Analysis + Amelogenin\ Gene\ Detection + Paternity\ Testing$$

- **Forensic DNA Databases:**

$$DNA\ Profiling\ Storage + CODIS\ (Combined\ DNA\ Index\ System) + Matching\ Algorithms$$

Understanding the techniques used in DNA profiling is essential for reliable and accurate forensic analysis in criminal investigations.

7.6　Mitochondrial DNA Analysis

Mitochondrial DNA (mtDNA) analysis is a specialized technique in forensic genetics. Let's simplify this using essential concepts:

- **mtDNA Extraction:**

  Isolation from Cells + Purification Techniques + Mitochondrial Fractionation

- **mtDNA Amplification:**

  Polymerase Chain Reaction (PCR) + mtDNA Specific Primers + Targeted Regions

- **Sanger Sequencing:**

  Dideoxy Chain Termination + Fluorescent Labeling + Electrophoresis

- **Haplogroup Determination:**

  Variant Analysis + Phylogenetic Tree Classification + Ancestral Lineage Assignment

- **Comparison and Matching:**

  mtDNA Profile Comparison + Sequence Alignment + Sequence Homology Assessment

- **Advantages of mtDNA Analysis:**

  Maternal Lineage Tracing + Higher Copy Numbers + Degraded or Limited Samples

- **Limitations of mtDNA Analysis:**

  Lower Discriminatory Power + Matrilineal Inheritance + Population-Specific Haplotypes

Understanding the methods and applications of mtDNA analysis is crucial for its effective use in forensic investigations.

7.7   Challenges in DNA Analysis

DNA analysis in forensics comes with various challenges. Let's simplify this using essential concepts:

- **Low DNA Quantity:**

  Effective PCR Amplification + Sensitivity Enhancements + Multiple Replicates

- **DNA Degradation:**

  Repair Mechanisms + Short Target Sequences + Advanced Extraction Techniques

- **Mixtures and Contaminations:**

  Mixture Deconvolution + Probabilistic Genotyping + Strict Laboratory Protocols

- **Sample Preservation:**

  Proper Storage Conditions + Preventing DNA Contamination + Avoiding Degradation

- **Complex Forensic Samples:**

  Touch DNA Analysis + Forensic Body Fluids Identification + Environmental Influences

- **Interpretation and Statistics:**

  Likelihood Ratios + Population Genetics Data + Validated Statistical Models

- **Legal and Ethical Issues:**

  Chain of Custody Maintenance + Consent and Privacy Concerns + Expert Witness Testimony

Navigating through these challenges requires a comprehensive approach, including advanced techniques and stringent protocols.

- **DNA Preservation Challenges:**

  Long-term Storage + Preventing Degradation + Technological Advances

- **Advancements in DNA Extraction:**

  Improved Techniques + Low-Copy Number Analysis + Ancient DNA Recovery

- **Retroactive DNA Profiling:**

  Post-Conviction Testing + Re-examining Evidence + Innocence Projects

- **Phenotypic Analysis:**

  Predicting Physical Traits + Ancestry Estimation + Facial Reconstruction

- **Familial DNA Searching:**

  Partial Matches + Identifying Relatives + Generating Leads

- **Cold Case Solvability Factors:**

  DNA Evidence Quality + Preserved Crime Scene Materials + Availability of Suspect Profiles

- **Public Awareness and Collaboration:**

  Media Campaigns + Community Involvement + Law Enforcement Collaboration

Harnessing the power of DNA technology plays a crucial role in re-examining cold cases, offering hope for justice and closure.

Chapter 8

Forensic Psychiatry

8.1   Introduction to Forensic Psychiatry

Forensic psychiatry blends mental health and legal principles. Let's simplify this using essential concepts:

- **Mental State Examination (MSE):**

    Assessment of Appearance, Behavior, Mood, Thought Process, and Cognitive Function

- **Insanity Defense Criteria:**

    M'Naghten Rule+Irresistible Impulse Test+Durham Rule+ALI (American Law Institute) Test

- **Competency to Stand Trial:**

    Understanding Legal Proceedings + Assisting in Own Defense + Rational Decision-Making

- **Risk Assessment Tools:**

    HCR-20 (Historical Clinical Risk-20)+SVR-20 (Structured Professional Judgment for Violence Risk)

- **Psychopathy Assessment:**

    PCL-R (Psychopathy Checklist-Revised)+Factor 1: Interpersonal/Affective+Factor 2: Lifestyle/Antisocial

- **Diminished Capacity:**

Impaired Mental State Impacting Criminal Responsibility+Partial Defense in Some Jurisdictions

- **Psychiatric Evaluation in Legal Context:**

Objective Assessment of Mental Health+

Documenting Clinical Observations + Providing Expert Opinions

Understanding the intersection of psychiatry and the legal system is vital in forensic psychiatry practice.

8.2   Criminal Responsibility

Understanding criminal responsibility in forensic psychiatry involves complex factors. Let's simplify this using essential concepts:

- **M'Naghten Rule for Insanity:**

Insanity = Defect of Reasoning + Disease of the Mind $\implies$ Not Knowing Right from Wrong

- **Irresistible Impulse Test:**

Loss of Control + Inability to Resist Impulses $\implies$ Diminished Responsibility

- **Durham Rule:**

Crime Result of Mental Disorder $\implies$ Not Liable if Mental Disorder Contributed

- **ALI (American Law Institute) Standard:**

Mental Disease or Defect+Lack of Substantial Capacity $\implies$ Lack of Criminal Responsibility

- **Diminished Capacity:**

Mental Impairment + Reduced Mental Capacity $\implies$ Reduced Criminal Responsibility

- **Competency to Stand Trial:**

  Understanding Legal Proceedings + Assisting in Own Defense $\implies$ Competent to Stand Trial

- **Risk Assessment Tools:**

  Actuarial Risk Assessment + Clinical Judgment + Violence Risk Appraisal Guide (VRAG)

Assessing criminal responsibility involves a nuanced examination of mental states, capacity, and the impact of mental disorders on an individual's actions.

8.3   Competency to Stand Trial

Evaluating competency to stand trial involves key considerations. Let's simplify this using essential concepts:

- **Legal Criteria for Competency:**

  Understanding Legal Proceedings + Assisting in Own Defense $\implies$ Competent to Stand Trial

- **Decisional Capacity:**

  Ability to Make Informed Decisions + Understanding Consequences + Communication Skills

- **Competency Assessment Tools:**

  MacArthur Competence Assessment Tool-Criminal Adjudication (MacCAT-CA)

- **Mental Disorders Impact on Competency:**

  Psychotic Disorders + Cognitive Impairment + Mood Disorders $\implies$ Potential Incompetency

- **Competency Restoration:**

  Psychoeducation + Medication Management + Therapeutic Interventions

- **Competency vs. Criminal Responsibility:**

  Competency Focuses on Trial Participation $\neq$ Criminal Responsibility for Past Actions

- **Legal Procedures for Incompetency:**

$$\text{Competency Hearings} + \text{Treatment Plans} + \text{Reevaluation Procedures}$$

Ensuring the competency of individuals to stand trial involves a thorough evaluation of cognitive and decision-making abilities.

8.4 Insanity Defense

The insanity defense involves complex legal and psychiatric considerations. Let's simplify this using essential concepts:

- **M'Naghten Rule for Insanity:**

$$\text{Insanity} = \text{Defect of Reasoning} + \text{Disease of the Mind} \implies \text{Not Knowing Right from Wrong}$$

- **Irresistible Impulse Test:**

$$\text{Loss of Control} + \text{Inability to Resist Impulses} \implies \text{Diminished Responsibility}$$

- **Durham Rule:**

$$\text{Crime Result of Mental Disorder} \implies \text{Not Liable if Mental Disorder Contributed}$$

- **ALI (American Law Institute) Standard:**

$$\text{Mental Disease or Defect} + \text{Lack of Substantial Capacity} \implies \text{Lack of Criminal Responsibility}$$

- **Diminished Capacity:**

$$\text{Mental Impairment} + \text{Reduced Mental Capacity} \implies \text{Reduced Criminal Responsibility}$$

- **Competency to Stand Trial:**

$$\text{Understanding Legal Proceedings} + \text{Assisting in Own Defense} \implies \text{Competent to Stand Trial}$$

- **Psychiatric Evaluation in Insanity Cases:**

$$\text{Establishing Mental State at Time of Offense}$$
$$+ \text{Documenting Mental Disorders} + \text{Assessing Legal Criteria}$$

The insanity defense requires a careful examination of the accused's mental state at the time of the alleged crime and adherence to specific legal standards.

8.5 Psychological Autopsy

Psychological autopsy is a comprehensive study of a person's life, mental state, and the circumstances leading to their death. Let's simplify this using essential concepts:

- **Purpose of Psychological Autopsy:**

  Understanding Factors Leading to Death+Identifying Mental Health Issues+Uncovering Motivations

- **Information Gathering:**

  Medical Records + Interviews with Family and Associates + Analysis of Personal Writings

- **Psychiatric Evaluation:**

  Assessment of Mental Health History+Identification of Psychopathologies+Substance Use Evaluation

- **Social and Environmental Factors:**

  Relationships + Stressors + Work and Financial Situation

- **Risk Assessment:**

  Identification of Suicidal or Homicidal Ideation+Previous Attempts+Access to Lethal Means

- **Forensic Implications:**

  Determining Cause and Manner of Death + Providing Insights for Legal Proceedings

  +Preventing Future Incidents

- **Ethical Considerations:**

  Respecting Privacy+Ensuring Confidentiality+Balancing Therapeutic and Investigative Goals

Psychological autopsy serves as a valuable tool in understanding the complex interplay of factors leading to a person's death, facilitating both forensic and preventive perspectives.

8.6   Risk Assessment

Risk assessment in forensic psychiatry involves evaluating potential harm and mitigating factors. Let's simplify this using essential concepts:

- **Actuarial Risk Assessment:**

$$\text{Statistical Models} + \text{Historical Data} + \text{Risk Factors} \implies \text{Quantitative Prediction}$$

- **Clinical Risk Assessment:**

$$\text{Professional Judgment} + \text{Structured Clinical Interviews} + \text{Dynamic Risk Factors}$$

- **Violence Risk Appraisal Guide (VRAG):**

$$\text{Scoring System} + \text{Criminological Variables} + \text{Historical Factors}$$

- **HCR-20 (Historical Clinical Risk Management):**

$$\text{Structured Professional Judgment} + \text{Historical, Clinical, and Risk Factors}$$

- **Dynamic Risk Factors:**

$$\text{Mental Health Status} + \text{Substance Abuse} + \text{Stressors and Coping Strategies}$$

- **Protective Factors:**

$$\text{Social Support} + \text{Stable Employment} + \text{Positive Coping Mechanisms}$$

- **Risk Communication:**

$$\text{Clear Communication of Assessment Results} + \text{Informed Decision-Making}$$

$$+ \text{Collaboration with Stakeholders}$$

Conducting effective risk assessments involves a combination of quantitative models, clinical judgment, and consideration of dynamic factors to enhance decision-making in forensic psychiatry.

8.7 Mental Health Laws

Understanding mental health laws is crucial for forensic psychiatrists. Let's simplify this using essential concepts:

- **Involuntary Commitment Criteria:**

  Danger to Self + Danger to Others + Grave Disability $\implies$ Involuntary Hospitalization

- **Parens Patriae Doctrine:**

  State as Parent+Protecting Individuals Unable to Care for Themselves+Balancing Individual Rights

- **Assisted Outpatient Treatment (AOT):**

  Court-Ordered Mental Health Treatment + Community-Based

  +For Individuals with Severe Mental Illness

- **Tarasoff Duty to Warn:**

  Duty to Warn + Foreseeable Harm to a Specific Person + Confidentiality Limitations

- **Gravely Disabled Standard:**

  Unable to Provide Basic Needs + Extreme Functional Impairment + Risk of Harm to Self

- **Emergency Psychiatric Holds:**

  Immediate Danger to Self or Others + Temporary Detention + Psychiatric Evaluation

- **Insanity Defense Standards:**

  Legal Criteria for Insanity + M'Naghten Rule + Irresistible Impulse Test

Navigating mental health laws involves assessing the balance between individual rights and public safety, particularly in situations of involuntary commitment and treatment.

8.8   Psychological Profiling

Psychological profiling plays a crucial role in understanding criminal behavior. Let's simplify this using essential concepts:

- **Offender Typologies:**

  Organized vs. Disorganized + Crime Scene Characteristics + Behavioral Traits

- **Criminal Signature:**

  Distinctive Features in Crimes + Symbolic Elements + Consistency Across Offenses

- **Geographic Profiling:**

  Spatial Patterns of Crimes + Distance Decay + Probability Models

- **Victimology:**

  Target Selection Criteria + Relationships Between Offender and Victim + Motivations

- **Criminal Investigative Analysis (CIA):**

  Behavioral Analysis Unit (BAU) + Crime Scene Analysis + Criminal Behavior Patterns

- **Serial Offender Profiling:**

  Linkage Analysis + Commonalities Across Crimes + Temporal and Spatial Patterns

- **Psychopathy Checklist (PCL-R):**

  Interpersonal, Affective, and Lifestyle Factors + Assessment of Psychopathic Traits

Psychological profiling involves analyzing crime scene behaviors, offender characteristics, and patterns to assist law enforcement in criminal investigations.

Chapter 9

Forensic Entomology

9.1   Introduction to Forensic Entomology

Forensic entomology involves the study of insects and their role in legal investigations. Let's simplify this using essential concepts:

- **Postmortem Interval (PMI) Calculation:**

$$\text{Time of Insect Colonization} = \text{Time of Death} - \text{Initial Insect Arrival Time}$$

- **Succession of Insects:**

$$\text{Blow Flies} \rightarrow \text{Flesh Flies} \rightarrow \text{Beetles} \rightarrow \text{Mites}$$

- **Temperature-Dependent Development:**

$$\text{Degree-Days} = \frac{T_{\text{average}} - T_{\text{base}}}{\text{Developmental Rate}}$$

- **Minimum Postmortem Interval:**

$$\text{Determining Earliest Time of Insect Activity} + \text{Temperature and Environmental Factors}$$

- **Entomotoxicology:**

$$\text{Analysis of Insects for Toxins} + \text{Chemical Analysis of Larvae}$$

- **Urban vs. Rural Insect Succession:**

  Differences in Insect Species and Arrival Times + Urbanization Impact on Decomposition

- **Blow Fly Life Cycle:**

$$\text{Egg} \rightarrow \text{Larva} \rightarrow \text{Pupa} \rightarrow \text{Adult}$$

Forensic entomology aids in estimating the time of death by studying the colonization and development of insects on human remains.

9.2   Insect Succession on Carrion

Understanding the sequence of insect colonization on carrion is crucial for estimating the postmortem interval. Let's simplify this using essential concepts:

- **Fresh Stage:**

  Blow Flies (*Calliphoridae*) $\rightarrow$ Flesh Flies (*Sarcophagidae*) $\rightarrow$ Green Bottle Flies (*Lucilia*)

- **Bloat Stage:**

  Predatory Beetles (*Dermestidae*) $\rightarrow$ Carrion Beetles (*Silphidae*)

- **Decay Stage:**

  Carrion Beetles $\rightarrow$ Cheese Skippers (*Piophilidae*) $\rightarrow$ Hide Beetles (*Trogidae*)

- **Post-Decay Stage:**

  Predatory Beetles $\rightarrow$ Mites (*Acarina*) $\rightarrow$ Ants (*Formicidae*)

- **Dry Stage:**

  Dermestid Beetles (*Dermestidae*) $\rightarrow$ Moths (*Lepidoptera*) $\rightarrow$ Predatory Beetles

- **Remains Stage:**

  Scavenging Insects $\rightarrow$ Detritivores $\rightarrow$ Final Decomposition Stages

- **Factors Influencing Succession:**

  Temperature, Humidity, and Environmental Conditions → Availability of Resources

Insect succession on carrion follows a predictable pattern, aiding forensic entomologists in estimating the time since death based on the presence and developmental stage of specific insect species.

9.3 Role of Insects in Death Investigation

Insects play a vital role in death investigations, providing valuable information about the postmortem interval and other forensic aspects. Let's simplify this using essential concepts:

- **Mortality Rate Estimation:**

  Insect Colonization Rate × Life Cycle Duration = Postmortem Interval Estimate

- **Species Succession:**

  Sequence of Insect Species Arrival → Succession Pattern → Estimation of Decomposition Stages

- **Temperature-Dependent Development:**

$$\text{Degree-Days} = \frac{T_{\text{average}} - T_{\text{base}}}{\text{Developmental Rate}}$$

- **Entomotoxicology:**

  Analysis of Insects for Toxins → Identification of Chemicals in Decomposing Tissues

- **Criminal Investigations:**

  Linking Crime Scenes → Identifying Movement of Remains → Providing Additional Forensic Evidence

- **Insect Evidence Preservation:**

  Collection and Preservation Techniques → Maintaining Species and Developmental Stage Information

- **Forensic Entomology in Court:**

  Expert Witness Testimony → Presenting Entomological Findings to Legal Authorities

The role of insects in death investigations extends beyond postmortem interval estimation, contributing valuable data to various forensic aspects and aiding investigators in solving crimes.

9.4   Forensic Arachnology

Forensic arachnology, the study of spiders and other arachnids in forensic investigations, contributes valuable information to the death investigation process. Let's simplify this using essential concepts:

- **Arachnid Presence and Succession:**

$$\text{Spiders} \rightarrow \text{Scorpions} \rightarrow \text{Pseudoscorpions} \rightarrow \text{Harvestmen}$$

- **Ecological Significance:**

$$\text{Arachnids as Decomposers} \rightarrow \text{Role in Carrion Ecosystems} \rightarrow \text{Influence on Insect Succession}$$

- **Web Analysis:**

$$\text{Web Structure and Design} \rightarrow \text{Identification of Spider Species} \rightarrow \text{Environmental Conditions}$$

- **Predatory Behavior:**

$$\text{Preying on Insects} \rightarrow \text{Impact on Insect Colonization Patterns} \rightarrow \text{Time Since Death Estimation}$$

- **Silk Analysis:**

$$\text{Silk Composition} \rightarrow \text{Identification of Spider Species} \rightarrow \text{Environmental Conditions}$$

- **Toxicology Significance:**

$$\text{Venom Analysis} \rightarrow \text{Presence of Toxins in Decomposing Tissues} \rightarrow \text{Entomotoxicology}$$

- **Climbing Patterns:**

$$\text{Identification of Vertical Movement on Remains} \rightarrow \text{Linking Crime Scenes} \rightarrow \text{Forensic Significance}$$

Forensic arachnology enhances the understanding of arachnid presence, behavior, and ecological interactions, providing valuable insights into the forensic investigation process.

9.5 Applications in Legal Cases

Forensic entomology finds various applications in legal cases, providing crucial evidence and insights. Let's simplify this using essential concepts:

- **Time of Death Estimation:**

$$\text{Postmortem Interval} = \frac{\text{Total Accumulated Degree-Days}}{\text{Insect Developmental Rate}}$$

- **Crime Scene Linkage:**

$$\text{Insect Species and Stages} \rightarrow \text{Movement of Remains} \rightarrow \text{Linking Crime Scenes}$$

- **Drug and Toxin Analysis:**

$$\text{Entomotoxicology} \rightarrow \text{Identification of Toxins and Drugs in Decomposing Tissues}$$

- **Geographical Origin:**

$$\text{Identification of Indigenous Insects} \rightarrow \text{Geographical Location of Death}$$

- **Criminal Investigations:**

$$\text{Insect Evidence in Court} \rightarrow \text{Expert Witness Testimony} \rightarrow \text{Strengthening Legal Cases}$$

- **Forensic Profiling:**

$$\text{Insect Succession Patterns} \rightarrow \text{Profiling Decomposition Stages} \rightarrow \text{Supporting Investigative Findings}$$

- **Victim Movement:**

$$\text{Insect Colonization Along Routes} \rightarrow \text{Estimation of Victim Movement} \rightarrow \text{Crime Reconstruction}$$

Forensic entomology serves as a powerful tool in legal cases, contributing to time of death estimation, crime scene linkage, and various other aspects crucial for investigations and legal proceedings.

9.6 Collection and Preservation of Entomological Evidence

Proper collection and preservation of entomological evidence are crucial for accurate forensic analysis. Let's simplify this using essential concepts:

- **Collection Techniques:**

    Handpicking → Use of Entomological Tools → Proper Documentation

- **Preservation Methods:**

    Ethanol Preservation → Freezing at -20°C → Drying and Mounting

- **Documentation Protocols:**

    Date and Time of Collection → Location Coordinates → Environmental Conditions

- **Entomological Kits:**

    Standardized Kits for Collection → Includes Tools and Preservation Materials

- **Packaging and Transport:**

    Use of Airtight Containers → Protection from Contamination → Secure Transportation

- **Documentation Software:**

    Digital Records for Each Specimen → Photographic Documentation → Data Accessibility

- **Quality Control Measures:**

    Regular Calibration of Tools → Verification of Collection Procedures

    → Minimizing Cross-Contamination

Effective collection and preservation of entomological evidence involve systematic techniques, proper documentation, and adherence to quality control measures, ensuring reliable results in forensic investigations.

9.7 Entomotoxicology

Entomotoxicology, the study of toxins in insects associated with decomposing remains, plays a crucial role in forensic investigations. Let's simplify this using essential concepts:

- **Toxin Uptake by Insects:**

  Toxin Concentration in Decomposing Tissues → Insect Feeding and Uptake → Entomotoxicology Analysis

- **Analysis Techniques:**

  Gas Chromatography-Mass Spectrometry (GC-MS)

  → Liquid Chromatography-Mass Spectrometry (LC-MS) → Identification of Toxins

- **Toxin Persistence in Insects:**

  Decay Rates of Toxins in Insect Tissues → Postmortem Interval Estimation → Forensic Significance

- **Correlation with Decomposition Stages:**

  Toxin Concentration Changes over Decomposition Stages →

  Linking Insect Data to Time Since Death → Enhanced PMI Estimation

- **Drug Metabolism in Insects:**

  Identification of Metabolites in Insects → Understanding Drug Metabolism Processes

  → Forensic Drug Analysis

- **Validation and Quality Control:**

  Standardized Protocols for Analysis → Quality Assurance in Entomotoxicology

  → Reliable Forensic Evidence

Entomotoxicology provides valuable insights into the presence and persistence of toxins in insects associated with decomposing remains, aiding in forensic investigations and time of death estimation.

9.8   Forensic Acarology

Forensic acarology, the study of mites and ticks in forensic investigations, provides valuable insights into decomposition processes and environmental conditions. Let's simplify this using essential concepts:

- **Mite and Tick Identification:**

  Morphological Characteristics → Species Identification → Linking Acarofauna to Decomposition

- **Ecological Significance:**

  Role in Decomposition Ecosystems → Influence on Insect Succession

  → Environmental Forensic Indicators

- **Mite and Tick Succession:**

  Successive Colonization Patterns → Time Since Death Estimation → Forensic Significance

- **Mite and Tick-Associated Toxins:**

  Toxin Presence in Mites and Ticks → Entomotoxicology Analysis

  → Linking Toxin Data to Decomposition Stages

- **Environmental Factors:**

  Humidity and Temperature Influence → Correlation with Mite and Tick Populations

  → Environmental Clues in Forensic Investigations

- **Molecular Techniques:**

  DNA Barcoding for Species Identification → Genetic Analysis of Mite and Tick Populations

  → Enhancing Forensic Accuracy

- **Climatic Changes Impact:**

  Acarofauna Responses to Climate Shifts → Predictive Tools in Forensic Ecology

  → Advancing Time of Death Estimation

Forensic acarology enriches forensic investigations by providing data on mite and tick presence, ecological roles, and their significance in decomposition processes and environmental conditions.

Chapter 10

Forensic Ballistics

- **Bullet Trajectory Analysis:**

  Trajectory Path $\rightarrow$ Impact Angle $\rightarrow$ Forensic Reconstruction

- **Firearm Identification:**

  Caliber Measurement $\rightarrow$ Rifling Characteristics $\rightarrow$ Unique Firearm Signatures

- **Bullet and Casing Matching:**

  Striation Patterns $\rightarrow$ Firing Pin Impressions $\rightarrow$ Toolmark Analysis

- **Gunpowder Residue Analysis:**

  Residue Distribution $\rightarrow$ GSR (Gunshot Residue) Analysis $\rightarrow$ Shooter Proximity Estimation

- **Bullet Velocity Calculations:**

  Distance Traveled $\rightarrow$ Time of Flight $\rightarrow$ Velocity Formulas

- **Bullet Penetration and Energy:**

  Penetration Depth $\rightarrow$ Energy Transfer $\rightarrow$ Stopping Power

- **Trajectory Reconstruction Equations:**

  Bullet Drop Calculations $\rightarrow$ Windage and Elevation Adjustments $\rightarrow$ Shooter Positioning

Forensic ballistics employs mathematical formulas and analysis techniques to reconstruct shooting incidents, identify firearms, and provide critical evidence in criminal investigations.

10.1   Firearm Types and Mechanisms

Understanding the types and mechanisms of firearms is crucial in forensic ballistics. Let's simplify this with key formulas and ideas:

- **Firearm Classification:**

  Caliber Measurement $\rightarrow$ Firearm Categorization $\rightarrow$ Identification Parameters

- **Rifling Characteristics:**

  Groove and Lands Measurements $\rightarrow$ Twist Rate Calculations $\rightarrow$ Bullet Spin

- **Action Types and Formulas:**

  Bolt Action $\rightarrow$ Lever Action $\rightarrow$ Semi-Automatic

- **Recoil Energy Equations:**

  Mass of Firearm $\rightarrow$ Velocity of Bullet $\rightarrow$ Recoil Formulas

- **Gas Laws in Semi-Automatics:**

  Gas Expansion $\rightarrow$ Gas Pressure $\rightarrow$ Automatic Action

- **Bullet Cartridge Design:**

  Case Length $\rightarrow$ Bullet Shape $\rightarrow$ Cartridge Functionality

- **Primer Ignition Mechanism:**

  Striker-Fired $\rightarrow$ Firing Pin Mechanism $\rightarrow$ Primer Ignition

Forensic ballistics relies on the analysis of firearm types, rifling characteristics, and mechanisms to identify weapons, determine shooting scenarios, and contribute to criminal investigations.

10.2 Bullet and Cartridge Case Examination

The examination of bullets and cartridge cases in forensic ballistics involves crucial analysis techniques and concepts. Let's simplify this using key formulas and ideas:

- **Striation Patterns Analysis:**

  Comparison of Striations → Identification of Matching Characteristics → Individual Firearm Attribution

- **Firing Pin Impressions:**

  Unique Firing Pin Marks → Toolmark Analysis → Firearm Identification

- **Toolmark Matching Equations:**

  Microscopic Examination → Bullet and Case Toolmarks → Matching Formulas

- **Bullet and Case Imaging Techniques:**

  Photographic Documentation → 3D Imaging → Enhanced Analysis

- **Cartridge Case Expansion Analysis:**

  Cartridge Case Dimensions → Pressure and Expansion Formulas → Firearm Specifics

- **Projectile Path Calculation:**

  Bullet Trajectory Reconstruction → Impact Angle Determination → Shooting Incident Recreation

- **Gunshot Residue Examination:**

  Residue Distribution Patterns → GSR (Gunshot Residue) Analysis → Shooter Proximity Estimation

Bullet and cartridge case examination in forensic ballistics utilizes mathematical formulas and advanced analysis techniques to attribute specific characteristics to individual firearms and reconstruct shooting incidents.

10.3 Bullet Trajectory Analysis

Bullet trajectory analysis is a critical aspect of forensic ballistics, helping reconstruct shooting incidents. Let's simplify this using key formulas and concepts:

- **Trajectory Path Calculation:**

$$\text{Trajectory Path} = \frac{V_0^2 \sin(2\theta)}{g}$$

  where V_0 is the initial velocity, θ is the launch angle, and g is the acceleration due to gravity.

- **Impact Angle Determination:**

$$\text{Impact Angle} = \arctan\left(\frac{V_0 \sin(\theta)t}{V_0 \cos(\theta) - gt}\right)$$

- **Time of Flight Calculation:**

$$\text{Time of Flight} = \frac{2V_0 \sin(\theta)}{g}$$

- **Reconstruction Equations:**

$$\text{Shooter Position} = \frac{gt^2}{2} + V_0 \sin(\theta)t$$

$$\text{Horizontal Distance} = V_0 \cos(\theta)t$$

- **Windage and Elevation Adjustments:**

$$\text{Adjustment} = \text{Trajectory Deviation} \times \text{Correction Factor}$$

- **Shooting Incident Recreation:**

$$\text{Recreate Incident Conditions} \rightarrow \text{Trajectory Calculation} \rightarrow \text{Position and Angle Determination}$$

Bullet trajectory analysis utilizes these formulas to determine the trajectory path, impact angle, and recreate shooting incidents, aiding investigators in understanding the dynamics of firearm-related events.

10.4 Gunshot Residue Analysis

Gunshot residue (GSR) analysis is crucial in forensic ballistics for identifying shooter proximity. Let's simplify this using key formulas and concepts:

- **Residue Distribution Patterns:**

$$\text{Residue Distribution} \rightarrow \text{Distance from Muzzle} \rightarrow \text{Shooter Proximity}$$

- **GSR (Gunshot Residue) Composition:**

$$\text{GSR Components} = \text{Lead, Barium, Antimony, etc.}$$

- **Particle Analysis:**

$$\text{Microscopic Examination} \rightarrow \text{Particle Size and Shape} \rightarrow \text{Distance Estimation}$$

- **Residue Dispersion Equations:**

$$\text{Dispersion Pattern} = \frac{Q}{4\pi r^2}$$

  where Q is the total quantity of GSR and r is the distance from the muzzle.

- **Shooter Proximity Estimation:**

$$\text{Proximity} = \text{Analyzing Residue Concentration and Distribution}$$

- **Collection and Preservation Techniques:**

$$\text{Collection Methods} \rightarrow \text{Preservation in Forensic Analysis}$$

- **Confirmation Methods:**

$$\text{Secondary Confirmation Tests} \rightarrow \text{Ensuring Accurate Results}$$

Gunshot residue analysis employs these formulas to determine shooter proximity, analyze residue composition, and aid in reconstructing the dynamics of a shooting incident in forensic investigations.

10.5 Firearm Identification

Firearm identification is a crucial process in forensic ballistics, involving the analysis of distinctive features. Let's simplify this using key formulas and concepts:

- **Striation Patterns Analysis:**

$$\text{Comparison of Striations} \rightarrow \text{Identification of Matching Characteristics}$$

$$\rightarrow \text{Individual Firearm Attribution}$$

- **Firing Pin Impressions:**

$$\text{Unique Firing Pin Marks} \rightarrow \text{Toolmark Analysis} \rightarrow \text{Firearm Identification}$$

- **Toolmark Matching Equations:**

$$\text{Microscopic Examination} \rightarrow \text{Bullet and Case Toolmarks} \rightarrow \text{Matching Formulas}$$

- **Firearm-Specific Characteristics:**

$$\text{Breechface Marks, Extractor and Ejector Marks, etc.} \rightarrow \text{Individual Firearm Attribution}$$

- **Firearm Database Comparison:**

$$\text{Comparison with Existing Firearm Databases} \rightarrow \text{Possible Matches} \rightarrow \text{Firearm Identification}$$

- **Statistical Methods:**

$$\text{Probability of Random Match} \rightarrow \text{Statistical Confidence in Firearm Identification}$$

- **Firearm Classification:**

$$\text{Caliber, Type, and Model Identification} \rightarrow \text{Narrowing Down Possibilities}$$

Firearm identification utilizes these formulas and methods to attribute specific characteristics to individual firearms, aiding investigators in linking firearms to crime scenes and incidents.

10.6 Toolmarks in Ballistics

Toolmarks play a crucial role in forensic ballistics for firearm identification and linkage to crime scenes. Let's simplify this using key formulas and concepts:

- **Toolmark Analysis:**

  Microscopic Examination $\rightarrow$ Comparison with Reference Toolmarks $\rightarrow$ Identification

- **Striation Patterns:**

  Analysis of Striation Patterns $\rightarrow$ Matching Characteristics $\rightarrow$ Toolmark Attribution

- **Surface Impressions:**

  Analysis of Surface Impressions $\rightarrow$ Tool Surface Characteristics $\rightarrow$ Identification

- **Toolmark Matching Equations:**

  Comparison Formulas for Striations and Impressions $\rightarrow$ Statistical Probability of Match

- **Firearm Toolmarks:**

  Firing Pin Impressions, Extractor and Ejector Marks, etc. $\rightarrow$ Individual Firearm Attribution

- **Tool Database Comparison:**

  Comparison with Existing Toolmark Databases $\rightarrow$ Possible Matches $\rightarrow$ Toolmark Identification

- **Statistical Confidence:**

  Probability of Random Match $\rightarrow$ Statistical Confidence in Toolmark Identification

Toolmarks in ballistics are analyzed using these formulas and methods, aiding investigators in linking tools to specific incidents and suspects.

10.7 Virtual Reconstruction in Ballistics

Virtual reconstruction in ballistics utilizes advanced technologies for crime scene analysis. Let's simplify this using key formulas and concepts:

- **3D Trajectory Analysis:**

$$\text{Utilizing 3D Coordinates} \rightarrow \text{Projectile Trajectory Reconstruction}$$

$$\rightarrow \text{Shooter Position and Angle Estimation}$$

- **Virtual Crime Scene Mapping:**

$$\text{Integration of Ballistic Data} \rightarrow \text{Creating Virtual Crime Scene Maps}$$

$$\rightarrow \text{Visualization for Investigators}$$

- **Bullet Path Reconstruction:**

$$\text{Analyzing Impact Points} \rightarrow \text{Reconstructing Bullet Paths} \rightarrow \text{Understanding Incident Dynamics}$$

- **Firearm Simulation Models:**

$$\text{Creating Virtual Firearm Models} \rightarrow \text{Simulating Bullet Trajectories}$$

$$\rightarrow \text{Comparison with Real-world Data}$$

- **Digital Evidence Integration:**

$$\text{Incorporating Digital Crime Scene Data} \rightarrow \text{Virtual Reconstruction Models}$$

$$\rightarrow \text{Enhanced Crime Scene Analysis}$$

- **Statistical Analysis:**

$$\text{Probabilistic Models} \rightarrow \text{Statistical Confidence in Virtual Reconstructions}$$

$$\rightarrow \text{Supporting Investigative Conclusions}$$

- **Virtual Reality Tools:**

$$\text{Utilizing VR for Crime Scene Walkthroughs} \rightarrow \text{Enhanced Understanding for Investigators}$$

Virtual reconstruction in ballistics employs these formulas and technologies to provide investigators with detailed insights into crime scene dynamics and assist in the reconstruction of shooting incidents.

Chapter 11

Digital Forensics

11.1 Introduction to Digital Forensics

Digital forensics is a critical field for investigating cybercrimes and analyzing electronic evidence. Let's simplify this using key formulas and concepts:

- **Data Recovery:**

  Deleted File Recovery Techniques $\rightarrow$ Hexadecimal Analysis $\rightarrow$ File Signature Identification

- **Disk Imaging:**

  Bit-for-Bit Copying of Storage Media $\rightarrow$ Creating Forensic Disk Images

  $\rightarrow$ Preserving Original Data Integrity

- **File Timestamp Analysis:**

  Interpreting Creation, Modification, and Access Timestamps

  $\rightarrow$ Timeline Reconstruction $\rightarrow$ Establishing Sequence of Events

- **Metadata Examination:**

  Analyzing File Metadata $\rightarrow$ Extracting Information on File Origins $\rightarrow$ Attribution and Context

- **Hash Functions:**

  MD5, SHA-1, SHA-256 Hashing $\rightarrow$ Data Integrity Verification

  $\rightarrow$ Digital Signatures and Verification

- **Network Forensics:**

  Capturing and Analyzing Network Traffic $\rightarrow$ Identifying Suspicious Patterns

  $\rightarrow$ Traceback and Attribution

- **Malware Analysis:**

  Behavioral Analysis $\rightarrow$ Signature-based Detection $\rightarrow$ Code Reverse Engineering

Digital forensics relies on these formulas and methods to uncover evidence, trace digital activities, and support investigations in the realm of cybercrime.

11.2   Computer and Mobile Device Analysis

Analyzing computers and mobile devices is fundamental in digital forensics. Let's simplify this using key formulas and concepts:

- **Storage Media Analysis:**

  Partition Table Examination $\rightarrow$ File System Analysis $\rightarrow$ Data Carving for Fragmented Files

- **Registry Forensics:**

  Analyzing Windows Registry Entries $\rightarrow$ Extracting System Configuration

  $\rightarrow$ User Activity Tracking

- **Mobile Device Extraction:**

  Logical, Physical, and File System Extraction $\rightarrow$ Decrypting Mobile Data

  $\rightarrow$ Recovering Deleted Messages and Call Logs

- **Cloud Forensics:**

  Accessing and Analyzing Cloud Storage $\rightarrow$ Metadata Examination

  $\rightarrow$ Linking Digital Activities to Cloud Services

- **Geolocation Analysis:**

  Interpreting GPS Coordinates $\rightarrow$ Mapping User Movements $\rightarrow$ Timeline of Device Locations

- **Communication Analysis:**

  Network Packet Inspection $\rightarrow$ Email Header Examination $\rightarrow$ Identifying Communication Patterns

- **Encryption and Decryption:**

  Breaking Encryption Algorithms $\rightarrow$ Password Cracking Techniques $\rightarrow$ Accessing Protected Data

Computer and mobile device analysis in digital forensics leverages these formulas and methodologies to extract valuable evidence and reconstruct digital activities.

11.3   File Systems and Data Recovery

Understanding file systems and data recovery is crucial in digital forensics. Let's simplify this using key formulas and concepts:

- **File System Structures:**

  Master File Table (MFT) for NTFS $\rightarrow$ Inode Table for Ext4 $\rightarrow$ FAT Table for FAT32

- **File Allocation Methods:**

  Contiguous Allocation $\rightarrow$ Linked Allocation $\rightarrow$ Indexed Allocation

- **Data Carving Techniques:**

  Header and Footer Signatures $\rightarrow$ Entropy Analysis for File Type Identification

  $\rightarrow$ Recovering Deleted Files

- **Data Recovery Tools:**

  dd (Disk Dump) $\rightarrow$ TestDisk and PhotoRec $\rightarrow$ Foremost for File Carving

- **RAID Recovery:**

  Parity Bit Analysis for RAID 5 $\rightarrow$ Rebuilding Striped Data $\rightarrow$ Ensuring Data Integrity

- **Journaling File Systems:**

  Journal Analysis for Ext3/Ext4 $\rightarrow$ Recovering Incomplete Transactions

  $\rightarrow$ Maintaining File System Consistency

- **Metadata Recovery:**

  Inode Information Recovery $\rightarrow$ Timestamp Reconstruction $\rightarrow$ Restoring File Attributes

File systems and data recovery in digital forensics rely on these formulas and methods to reconstruct file structures, retrieve lost data, and analyze storage media effectively.

11.4   Network Forensics

Network forensics plays a vital role in uncovering digital evidence related to cybercrimes. Let's simplify this using key formulas and concepts:

- **Packet Analysis:**

  Capturing Network Traffic (Sniffing) $\rightarrow$ Packet Header Inspection $\rightarrow$ Payload Extraction

- **Protocol Analysis:**

  Identifying Protocols (TCP, UDP, ICMP) $\rightarrow$ Session Reconstruction $\rightarrow$ Flow Pattern Analysis

- **Timestamp Analysis:**

  Coordinated Universal Time (UTC) $\rightarrow$ Network Time Protocol (NTP)

  $\rightarrow$ Aligning Timestamps for Events

- **Traffic Pattern Recognition:**

$$\text{Normal vs. Anomalous Patterns} \rightarrow \text{Statistical Analysis of Traffic}$$

$$\rightarrow \text{Detecting Intrusion or Malicious Activity}$$

- **DNS Forensics:**

$$\text{Resolving Domain Names} \rightarrow \text{Analyzing DNS Query Logs} \rightarrow \text{Identifying Suspicious Domain Activity}$$

- **IP Address Analysis:**

$$\text{Geolocation of IP Addresses} \rightarrow \text{Identifying Source and Destination IP}$$

$$\rightarrow \text{Correlating IP Addresses with Known Threats}$$

- **Network Security Protocols:**

$$\text{SSL/TLS Encryption Analysis} \rightarrow \text{Detecting Malicious Payloads} \rightarrow \text{Analyzing Encrypted Communication}$$

Network forensics uses these formulas and methodologies to analyze network traffic, detect anomalies, and reconstruct digital events for investigative purposes.

11.5 Cybercrime Investigations

Cybercrime investigations involve complex processes to uncover digital evidence related to online criminal activities. Let's simplify this using key formulas and concepts:

- **Incident Response Framework:**

$$\text{Preparation} \rightarrow \text{Identification} \rightarrow \text{Containment} \rightarrow \text{Eradication} \rightarrow \text{Recovery}$$

- **Digital Evidence Seizure:**

$$\text{Chain of Custody} \rightarrow \text{Forensic Imaging} \rightarrow \text{Write-Blockers} \rightarrow \text{Preserving Evidence Integrity}$$

- **Volatility Analysis:**

$$\text{Memory Forensics} \rightarrow \text{Identifying Running Processes} \rightarrow \text{Extracting Artifacts from RAM}$$

- **Malware Analysis:**

  Static Analysis → Dynamic Analysis → Behavioral Analysis → Signature-Based Detection

- **Cryptocurrency Tracing:**

  Blockchain Analysis → Transaction Linking → Identifying Wallet Addresses

  → Tracking Financial Flows

- **Network Forensic Analysis:**

  Packet Inspection → Log Analysis → Traffic Pattern Recognition → IP Address Attribution

- **Legal Considerations:**

  Chain of Custody Compliance → Admissibility of Digital Evidence

  → Courtroom Presentation of Findings

Cybercrime investigations use these formulas and methodologies to respond to incidents, seize digital evidence, analyze malware, trace cryptocurrency transactions, conduct network forensics, and comply with legal requirements.

11.6   Forensic Analysis of Malware

Forensic analysis of malware involves intricate processes to dissect malicious software and understand its behavior. Let's simplify this using key formulas and concepts:

- **Static Analysis:**

  File Header Analysis → Code Obfuscation Detection

  → Signature Matching → API Function Call Analysis

- **Dynamic Analysis:**

  Behavioral Monitoring → Sandbox Execution

  → Network Activity Analysis → Memory Analysis

- **Code Analysis:**

  Disassembly $\rightarrow$ Decompilation $\rightarrow$ Control Flow Analysis $\rightarrow$ Data Flow Analysis

- **Hashing Techniques:**

  MD5 $\rightarrow$ SHA-1 $\rightarrow$ SHA-256 $\rightarrow$ Checksum Calculations

- **Cryptanalysis for Encrypted Malware:**

  Brute-Force Attacks $\rightarrow$ Frequency Analysis $\rightarrow$ Known-Plaintext Attacks $\rightarrow$ Key Recovery

- **Timeline Analysis:**

  Creation Time $\rightarrow$ Modification Time $\rightarrow$ Last Accessed Time $\rightarrow$ Timeline Reconstruction

- **Cross-Matching with Threat Intelligence:**

  Indicator of Compromise (IoC) Matching $\rightarrow$ YARA Rule Application

  $\rightarrow$ Behavior Correlation with Known Threats

- **Reporting and Documentation:**

  Detailed Analysis Report $\rightarrow$ Recommendations for Mitigation

  $\rightarrow$ Sharing Findings with Cybersecurity Community

Forensic analysis of malware uses these formulas and methodologies to conduct static and dynamic analyses, understand code behavior, apply hashing techniques, decrypt encrypted malware, analyze timelines, and cross-match findings with threat intelligence.

11.7 Digital Evidence Handling

Effective digital evidence handling is crucial for maintaining the integrity of data. Let's simplify this using key formulas and concepts:

- **Chain of Custody:**

  Chain of Custody (CoC) = Documented Procedures $\rightarrow$ Secure Storage $\rightarrow$ Access Logs

- **Hashing for Integrity:**

$$\text{Hash Value} = \text{Hashing Algorithm}(\text{Digital Evidence})$$

- **Encryption for Confidentiality:**

$$\text{Encrypted Data} = \text{Encryption Algorithm}(\text{Digital Evidence})$$

- **Time Stamping:**

$$\text{Timestamp} = \text{Time Synchronization}(\text{System Clock})$$

- **Write-Blocking:**

$$\text{Write-Blocked Access} = \text{Write-Blocking Device}(\text{Storage Media})$$

- **Forensic Imaging:**

$$\text{Forensic Image} = \text{Bit-by-Bit Copy}(\text{Storage Media})$$

- **Metadata Preservation:**

$$\text{Metadata} = \text{Preserve File Attributes, Timestamps, and Ownership}$$

- **Forensic Tools Validation:**

$$\text{Tool Validation} = \text{Comparison with Known Results} \rightarrow \text{Verification of Integrity}$$

- **Secure Transfer:**

$$\text{Encrypted Transmission} = \text{Secure Protocols}(\text{Digital Evidence Transfer})$$

- **Documentation:**

$$\text{Detailed Log} = \text{Record of Actions} \rightarrow \text{Documentation of Findings}$$

Digital evidence handling relies on these formulas and methodologies to maintain a secure chain of custody, ensure data integrity through hashing, preserve confidentiality with encryption, timestamp events, implement write-blocking, create forensic images, preserve metadata, validate forensic tools, securely transfer evidence, and maintain comprehensive documentation.

11.8   Legal Issues in Digital Forensics

Navigating the legal landscape in digital forensics involves understanding key concepts and principles. Let's simplify this using essential formulas and considerations:

- **Legal Admissibility:**

$$\text{Admissible Evidence} = \text{Legally Obtained Evidence} \rightarrow \text{Proper Documentation}$$

- **Chain of Custody in Legal Context:**

$$\text{Legal CoC} = \text{Validated Procedures} \rightarrow \text{Court-Admissible Logs}$$

- **Authentication of Digital Evidence:**

$$\text{Digital Evidence Authentication} = \text{Hash Value Verification} \rightarrow \text{Expert Testimony}$$

- **Expert Witness Testimony:**

$$\text{Effective Testimony} = \text{Technical Competence} \rightarrow \text{Clear Communication}$$

- **Fourth Amendment Considerations:**

$$\text{Legal Search \& Seizure} = \text{Reasonable Expectation of Privacy} \rightarrow \text{Warrant Requirements}$$

- **Data Privacy Laws Compliance:**

$$\text{Compliance} = \text{Digital Forensics Procedures} \rightarrow \text{Data Protection Laws}$$

- **E-Discovery Rules:**

$$\text{Effective E-Discovery} = \text{Preservation} \rightarrow \text{Relevance and Proportionality}$$

- **Legal Documentation:**

$$\text{Legal Reports} = \text{Comprehensive Documentation} \rightarrow \text{Legal Language}$$

- **Ethical Considerations:**

$$\text{Ethical Conduct} = \text{Professional Integrity} \rightarrow \text{Respect for Privacy}$$

- **Data Destruction Compliance:**

$$\text{Secure Data Disposal} = \text{Legal Compliance} \rightarrow \text{Permanent Data Erasure}$$

Understanding the legal aspects of digital forensics involves adhering to these formulas and considerations, ensuring the admissibility of evidence, maintaining a legal chain of custody, authenticating digital evidence, providing expert testimony, respecting privacy rights, complying with data protection laws, following e-discovery rules, producing legal documentation, upholding ethical standards, and ensuring secure data disposal in compliance with legal requirements.

Chapter 12

Forensic Toxicology

12.1   Introduction to Toxicology

Toxicology is the study of the adverse effects of chemicals on living organisms. Let's simplify this introduction with key formulas and concepts:

- **Dose-Response Relationship:**

$$\text{Response} = f(\text{Dose})$$

- **LD50 Calculation:**

$$\text{LD50} = \frac{\text{Median Lethal Dose}}{\text{Body Weight of Test Animals}}$$

- **Absorption Rate:**

$$\text{Absorption Rate} = \frac{\text{Amount Absorbed}}{\text{Time}}$$

- **Distribution Coefficient:**

$$\text{Distribution Coefficient (D)} = \frac{\text{Concentration in Tissue}}{\text{Concentration in Blood}}$$

- **Metabolism Rate:**

$$\text{Metabolism Rate} = \frac{\text{Rate of Metabolism}}{\text{Initial Concentration}}$$

- **Excretion Rate:**

$$\text{Excretion Rate} = \frac{\text{Rate of Excretion}}{\text{Initial Concentration}}$$

- **Half-Life Calculation:**

$$\text{Half-Life}(t_{1/2}) = \frac{0.693}{\text{Elimination Rate Constant}}$$

- **Bioavailability:**

$$\text{Bioavailability} = \frac{\text{Amount of Drug Reaching Systemic Circulation}}{\text{Total Amount Administered}}$$

- **Toxicokinetics:**

$$\text{Toxicokinetics} = \text{Absorption} \rightarrow \text{Distribution} \rightarrow \text{Metabolism} \rightarrow \text{Excretion}$$

- **Toxicodynamics:**

$$\text{Toxicodynamics} = \text{Interaction with Target Molecules} \rightarrow \text{Cellular Response} \rightarrow \text{Adverse Effects}$$

Understanding toxicology involves exploring these formulas, including dose-response relationships, LD50 calculations, absorption rates, distribution coefficients, metabolism and excretion rates, half-life calculations, bioavailability, and the processes of toxicokinetics and toxicodynamics.

12.2   Classes of Poisons

Forensic toxicology categorizes poisons into various classes based on their chemical nature and effects. Let's explore these classes with key formulas and concepts:

- **Heavy Metals:**

$$\text{Heavy Metal Poisoning} = f(\text{Exposure Time}, \text{Concentration})$$

- **Alcohols:**

$$\text{Blood Alcohol Concentration (BAC)} = \frac{\text{Alcohol Absorbed}}{\text{Body Fluid Volume}}$$

- **Opioids:**

$$\text{Opioid Toxicity} = f(\text{Dose}, \text{Tolerance}, \text{Dependence})$$

- **Sedatives and Hypnotics:**

$$\text{Sedative Overdose Risk} = f(\text{Dosage}, \text{Body Weight})$$

- **Stimulants:**

$$\text{Stimulant Toxicity} = f(\text{Dose}, \text{Individual Sensitivity})$$

- **Hallucinogens:**

$$\text{Hallucinogenic Effects} = f(\text{Chemical Structure}, \text{Dose})$$

- **Toxic Gases:**

$$\text{Toxic Gas Exposure} = f(\text{Concentration}, \text{Duration})$$

- **Pesticides:**

$$\text{Pesticide Toxicity} = f(\text{Chemical Structure}, \text{Exposure Route})$$

- **Plant Toxins:**

$$\text{Plant Poisoning Severity} = f(\text{Toxin Concentration}, \text{Ingested Amount})$$

- **Chemical Warfare Agents:**

$$\text{Toxicity of Chemical Warfare Agents} = f(\text{Exposure Time}, \text{Concentration})$$

Understanding the classes of poisons involves exploring these formulas, including heavy metal poisoning factors, alcohol absorption rates, opioid toxicity factors, sedative and hypnotic overdose risks, stimulant toxicity factors, hallucinogenic effects, toxic gas exposure factors, pesticide toxicity factors, plant toxin poisoning severity, and the toxicity of chemical warfare agents.

12.3 Methods of Toxicological Analysis

Toxicological analysis plays a crucial role in identifying and quantifying toxins present in biological samples. Let's delve into the methods and key formulas used in toxicological analysis:

- **Gas Chromatography (GC):**

$$\text{Retention Time (RT)} = f(\text{Temperature}, \text{Mobile Phase Composition})$$

- **Liquid Chromatography (LC):**

$$\text{Retention Time (RT)} = f(\text{Column Type}, \text{Mobile Phase})$$

- **Mass Spectrometry (MS):**

$$\text{Mass-to-Charge Ratio (m/z)} = f(\text{Ionization Source}, \text{Detector Type})$$

- **Enzyme-Linked Immunosorbent Assay (ELISA):**

$$\text{Concentration of Analyte} = f(\text{Colorimetric Absorbance}, \text{Calibration Curve})$$

- **Polymerase Chain Reaction (PCR):**

$$\text{Amplification Factor} = f(\text{Number of Cycles}, \text{Primer Efficiency})$$

- **Thin-Layer Chromatography (TLC):**

$$\text{Rf Value} = f(\text{Solvent System}, \text{Stationary Phase})$$

- **Immunoassays:**

$$\text{Binding Affinity} = f(\text{Antigen-Antibody Interaction}, \text{Assay Sensitivity})$$

- **Nuclear Magnetic Resonance (NMR):**

$$\text{Chemical Shift} = f(\text{Magnetic Field Strength}, \text{Sample Composition})$$

Understanding the methods of toxicological analysis involves exploring these formulas, including retention time in chromatography, mass-to-charge ratio in mass spectrometry, concentration determination in ELISA, amplification factor in PCR, Rf value in TLC, binding affinity in immunoassays, and chemical shift in NMR.

12.4 Drug Metabolism

Understanding drug metabolism is vital in forensic toxicology to assess how the body processes and eliminates drugs. Let's explore the key aspects of drug metabolism and associated formulas:

- **First-Order Metabolism:**

$$\text{Rate of Metabolism} = k \times \text{Concentration of Drug}$$

- **Zero-Order Metabolism:**

$$\text{Rate of Metabolism} = k$$

- **Half-Life (t½):**

$$t_{\frac{1}{2}} = \frac{0.693}{k}$$

- **Clearance (Cl):**

$$\text{Cl} = \frac{\text{Dose}}{\text{Area under the Plasma Concentration-Time Curve (AUC)}}$$

- **Volume of Distribution (Vd):**

$$\text{Vd} = \frac{\text{Amount of Drug in the Body}}{\text{Concentration of Drug in Plasma}}$$

- **Bioavailability (F):**

$$F = \frac{\text{Area under the Oral Plasma Concentration-Time Curve (AUC)}}{\text{Area under the Intravenous Plasma Concentration-Time Curve (AUC)}}$$

- **Metabolic Pathways:**

$$\text{Metabolite Formation} = f(\text{Enzymes involved}, \text{Chemical Reactions})$$

These formulas provide insights into drug metabolism kinetics, including first-order and zero-order processes, half-life, clearance, volume of distribution, bioavailability, and the various metabolic pathways involved.

12.5   Postmortem Redistribution

Postmortem redistribution is a crucial consideration in forensic toxicology, impacting the accurate interpretation of drug levels. Let's explore the key aspects of postmortem redistribution and associated formulas:

- **Postmortem Redistribution Factor (PRF):**

$$\text{PRF} = \frac{\text{Concentration in Peripheral Blood}}{\text{Concentration in Central Blood (Heart)}}$$

- **Correction for Postmortem Redistribution:**

$$\text{Corrected Concentration} = \frac{\text{Peripheral Blood Concentration}}{\text{PRF}}$$

- **Limitations and Factors Influencing PRF:**

$$\text{PRF} = f(\text{Time Since Death}, \text{Drug Properties}, \text{Body Conditions})$$

- **Importance of Sampling Sites:**

$$\text{Appropriate Sampling Sites} = f(\text{Drug Characteristics}, \text{Body Conditions})$$

These formulas provide insights into postmortem redistribution factors, corrections for accurate drug concentration assessment, and the influencing factors that need consideration during forensic toxicological analysis.

12.6 Toxicological Interpretation

Toxicological interpretation in forensic toxicology involves assessing the significance of detected substances in relation to potential harm. Let's explore key concepts and formulas for toxicological interpretation:

- **Therapeutic Index (TI):**

$$\text{TI} = \frac{\text{Lethal Dose (LD)}}{\text{Effective Dose (ED)}}$$

- **Margin of Safety (MOS):**

$$\text{MOS} = \frac{\text{Therapeutic Dose} - \text{Toxic Dose}}{\text{Toxic Dose}}$$

- **LD50 and ED50:**

$$\text{LD50} - \text{Dose at which 50\% of the population is lethal}$$

$$\text{ED50} - \text{Dose at which 50\% of the population shows the desired effect}$$

- **Metabolic Pathways and Metabolite Identification:**

$$\text{Parent Compound} \xrightarrow{\text{Metabolic Enzymes}} \text{Metabolite 1, Metabolite 2, ...}$$

- **Toxicokinetics:**

$$C = \frac{\text{Dose}}{\text{Clearance Rate}}$$

- **Threshold Limit Value (TLV) and Biological Exposure Index (BEI):**

$$\text{TLV} \quad \text{BEI} = f(\text{Biological Samples})$$

These formulas aid in evaluating the potential toxicity of substances, understanding dose-response relationships, and interpreting toxicological findings in forensic investigations.

12.7 Case Studies

Let's delve into real-world applications of forensic toxicology through illustrative case studies. In each case, we'll highlight key toxicological findings and relevant formulas:

12.7.1 Case 1:

A victim is found deceased, and toxicological analysis reveals the presence of a substance. Key formulas include:

- **Blood-Alcohol Concentration (BAC):**

$$\text{BAC} = \frac{\text{Amount of Alcohol}}{\text{Blood Volume}}$$

- **Half-Life ($T_{1/2}$):**

$$T_{1/2} = \frac{\ln(2)}{\text{Elimination Rate}}$$

- **Toxicology Screen Results:**

$$\text{Positive/Negative for Substance X}$$

12.7.2 Case 2:

A suspicious death involving multiple substances prompts a detailed toxicological examination. Formulas include:

- **Polydrug Toxicity Assessment:**

$$\text{LD50 Combination} = \sum \text{LD50 Individual Substances}$$

- **Synergistic Effects:**

$$\text{Effect of Combined Substances} > \sum \text{Individual Effects}$$

- **Metabolic Interactions:**

$$\text{Interaction Potential} = \text{Metabolite 1} + \text{Metabolite 2}$$

These case studies showcase the practical application of forensic toxicology principles in unraveling complex scenarios.

12.8 Forensic Pharmacology

Explore the intersection of pharmacology and forensic science, uncovering the impact of drugs on forensic investigations.

- **Absorption Rate (AR):**

$$AR = \frac{\text{Amount Absorbed}}{\text{Time}}$$

- **Distribution Volume (Vd):**

$$Vd = \frac{\text{Amount of Drug in the Body}}{\text{Concentration in Plasma}}$$

- **Elimination Rate (ER):**

$$ER = \frac{\ln(2)}{\text{Half-Life}}$$

- **Pharmacokinetic Equations:**

$$C = \frac{D}{Vd \cdot \text{bioavailability}}$$

- **Enzyme-Inducing Potential:**

$$\text{Potential} = \text{Inducing Drug A} + \text{Inducing Drug B}$$

- **Drug-Drug Interactions:**

$$\text{Interaction Potential} = \text{Effect of Drug X} + \text{Effect of Drug Y}$$

Incorporate these formulas to decipher the pharmacological aspects of forensic cases, shedding light on drug behavior within the human body.

Chapter 13

Forensic Serology and DNA Analysis

13.1 Blood and Bloodstains

Unveil the secrets hidden in blood and bloodstains, essential elements in forensic serology and DNA analysis.

- **Blood Typing:** Understand the ABO and Rh blood group systems for individual identification.

- **Bloodstain Pattern Analysis (BPA):** Decode crime scenes through the examination of bloodstain patterns.

- **Angle of Impact (θ):**

$$\sin(\theta) = \frac{\text{Drop's Width}}{\text{Drop's Length}}$$

- **Area of Convergence:** Pinpoint the location of the blood source.

- **Luminol Reaction:** Illuminate blood traces in low-light conditions.

Chemical reaction: $3\,C_8H_7N_3O_2 + 3\,H_2O_2 + \text{blood hemoglobin} \xrightarrow{\text{catalyst}} \text{chemiluminescence}$

- **Presumptive Tests:** Leverage Kastle-Meyer, Hemastix, or Luminol tests for quick blood detection.

- **DNA Extraction from Blood:** Utilize specific protocols for isolating DNA from blood samples.

Empower your forensic investigations by mastering the intricacies of blood analysis, unraveling crucial details for justice.

13.2   Blood Group Systems

Uncover the genetic codes inscribed in blood through key blood group systems for forensic serology.

- **ABO Blood Group System:** Decode the A, B, and O blood types with the following inheritance rule:

$$\text{Blood Type} = \text{Alleles inherited from parents } (I^A, I^B, \text{ or } i)$$

- **Rh Blood Group System:** Navigate the positive (+) or negative (-) Rh factor inherited as a dominant trait.

- **MN Blood Group System:** Explore the M and N antigens, adding nuance to blood typing.

- **Lewis Blood Group System:** Investigate the presence or absence of Le^a and Le^b antigens.

- **Duffy Blood Group System:** Probe the Fy^a and Fy^b antigens for a more comprehensive blood profile.

- **Kell Blood Group System:** Unravel the intricacies of the Kell system with K and k antigens.

- **Diego Blood Group System:** Delve into the Diego system marked by Di^a and Di^b antigens.

- **Xg Blood Group System:** Illuminate the Xg system, contributing to gender-based distinctions.

- **Indian Blood Group System:** Recognize the significance of In^a and In^b antigens.

Unlock the mysteries encoded in blood group systems, providing vital information in forensic investigations.

13.3 DNA Structure and Function

Unveil the fundamental architecture and dynamic functions of DNA, the blueprint of life.

- **Double Helix Structure:** Envision the iconic double helix, a spiraled ladder comprising paired nucleotide rungs.

- **Nucleotide Composition:** Dissect a nucleotide—phosphate, deoxyribose sugar, and nitrogenous base (adenine, thymine, cytosine, or guanine).

- **Base Pairing Rules:** Decipher the code—adenine pairs with thymine, and cytosine pairs with guanine, united by hydrogen bonds.

- **Antiparallel Orientation:** Grasp the antiparallel arrangement of DNA strands, critical for replication and transcription.

- **DNA Replication:** Illuminate the duplication process where DNA unwinds, and new strands form based on complementary base pairing.

- **Transcription:** Decode the conversion of DNA instructions into RNA, facilitated by RNA polymerase.

- **Translation:** Witness the transformation of RNA into proteins, guided by ribosomes and transfer RNA.

- **Genetic Code:** Delve into the language of DNA, where three-nucleotide codons encode specific amino acids.

- **Role in Forensics:** Recognize DNA as a forensic powerhouse, providing unique identifiers through DNA profiling.

Embark on a journey through the intricate world of DNA, where structure meets function, shaping the landscape of forensic analysis.

13.4 Forensic DNA Typing

Uncover the world of Forensic DNA Typing—a key player in solving mysteries. Let's navigate through its core concepts:

- **PCR (Polymerase Chain Reaction):** Visualize the DNA amplification magic—PCR exponentially replicates targeted DNA regions.

- **Short Tandem Repeats (STRs):** Grasp the significance of STRs—short, repetitive DNA sequences with unique variations among individuals.

- **Electrophoresis:** Witness the separation of DNA fragments based on size using gel electrophoresis, creating distinct banding patterns.

- **DNA Profiling:** Comprehend the creation of a DNA profile—unique to each individual due to the combination of their STR patterns.

- **Capillary Electrophoresis:** Upgrade the technique to capillary electrophoresis, enhancing speed and precision in separating DNA fragments.

- **Amelogenin Gene:** Identify the gender marker—Amelogenin gene distinguishes X and Y chromosomes, aiding sex determination.

- **Forensic Significance:** Embrace the role of Forensic DNA Typing in criminal investigations, paternity testing, and mass disaster victim identification.

In the realm of Forensic DNA Typing, each fragment tells a unique story, contributing to the unraveling of mysteries.

13.5 DNA Profiling Techniques

Embark on the journey through DNA profiling, a powerhouse in forensic investigations. Let's delve into its core techniques:

- **Polymerase Chain Reaction (PCR):** Envision the DNA amplification marvel—PCR rapidly replicates targeted DNA regions, unlocking a wealth of genetic information.

- **Short Tandem Repeats (STRs):** Grasp the essence of STRs—short, repetitive DNA sequences that exhibit unique variations among individuals, forming the basis for DNA profiling.

- **Gel Electrophoresis:** Witness the separation of DNA fragments by size using gel electrophoresis, creating distinctive patterns crucial for profiling.

- **Capillary Electrophoresis:** Elevate the process with capillary electrophoresis, enhancing the efficiency and precision of DNA fragment separation.

- **DNA Fragment Analysis:** Understand the analysis of DNA fragments to decipher individual profiles, each as distinctive as a fingerprint.

- **Genetic Markers:** Explore the role of genetic markers—unique regions in the genome used to differentiate individuals.

- **Forensic Applications:** Recognize the applications of DNA profiling in solving crimes, establishing paternity, and identifying victims in mass disasters.

In the realm of DNA profiling techniques, the language of genes speaks volumes, aiding forensic experts in solving the most intricate puzzles.

13.6   Mitochondrial DNA Analysis

Embark on the journey of mitochondrial DNA (mtDNA) analysis, a fascinating avenue in forensic genetics. Let's unravel its intricacies:

- **Mitochondrial DNA Overview:** Picture the powerhouse of the cell—the mitochondrion. Within, mtDNA reigns supreme, with unique properties and maternal inheritance.

- **Maternal Lineage Tracing:** Trace ancestry through the maternal line, as mtDNA is passed down from mother to offspring, offering insights into heritage.

- **Hypervariable Regions:** Dive into hypervariable regions, specific segments of mtDNA with heightened variability, acting as forensic goldmines.

- **mtDNA Sequencing:** Envision the sequencing process, decoding the order of nucleotides in mtDNA, a key step in the analysis.

- **Forensic Significance:** Grasp the forensic significance of mtDNA, especially in cases where nuclear DNA analysis may be challenging or unavailable.

- **Challenges and Limitations:** Acknowledge the challenges—lower discrimination power compared to nuclear DNA and complexities in interpretation.

- **Applications in Cold Cases:** Explore how mtDNA analysis shines in cold cases, where degraded or limited DNA samples find a voice in forensic investigations.

In the world of mitochondrial DNA analysis, the maternally inherited code unveils stories that endure across generations, aiding forensic detectives in their quest for truth.

13.7   Challenges in DNA Analysis

Embark on a journey through the challenges encountered in the intricate realm of DNA analysis:

- **Low DNA Quantity:** Imagine the hurdle of scarce DNA samples. Overcome this challenge with sensitive techniques like PCR amplification.

- **Degraded DNA:** Visualize the struggle when DNA degrades over time. Mitigate this obstacle by employing advanced extraction and amplification methods.

- **Contamination Concerns:** Picture the anxiety of contamination. Safeguard against it with rigorous laboratory practices and stringent protocols.

- **Complex Mixtures:** Navigate the complexity of mixed DNA samples. Employ sophisticated statistical algorithms to untangle the genetic web.

- **Inhibitors in Samples:** Confront inhibitors hindering DNA analysis. Counteract their effects through purification steps and innovative protocols.

- **Technological Limitations:** Acknowledge the limitations of current technologies. Anticipate breakthroughs for enhanced resolution and accuracy.

- **Interpretation Ambiguities:** Confront interpretation challenges. Apply expertise and constantly refine methodologies to reduce ambiguities.

In the face of these challenges, forensic DNA analysts stand resilient, adapting and innovating to extract truth from the genetic code.

13.8   Cold Cases and DNA

Unlock the mysteries of unresolved cases as DNA takes center stage:

- **DNA Time Capsules:** Envision DNA as a time-traveling detective. In cold cases, preserved DNA becomes a silent witness, waiting for the right technology to unveil its secrets.

- **Advancements in DNA Technologies:** Imagine the leap from the past to the present. Modern DNA analysis techniques, like STR profiling and mitochondrial DNA sequencing, breathe life into dormant cases.

- **Genetic Genealogy Revolution:** Picture a genealogical map guiding investigations. Genetic genealogy, powered by DNA databases, redefines family trees, unearthing connections and solving long-standing mysteries.

- **Familial DNA Searching:** Navigate the ethical landscape of familial DNA searching. Uncover leads by identifying relatives, bringing investigators closer to solving cases.

- **Isotopic Analysis:** Visualize isotopes revealing geographical secrets. This multidisciplinary approach, combined with DNA analysis, provides a holistic view, reconstructing the stories of unidentified victims.

In the realm of cold cases, DNA emerges as the key, transcending time to deliver justice.

Chapter 14

Forensic Anthropology

14.1 Bone Identification

Unravel the secrets hidden in bones with a glance:

- **Osteology Insights:** Dive into the structure of bones. Osteons, the fundamental units, hold the key to age and health assessment.

- **Morphological Clues:** Visualize the uniqueness in bone shapes. From the robusticity of the femur to the delicacy of the phalanges, each bone tells a distinctive tale.

- **Epiphyseal Fusion:** Decode age secrets through epiphyses. Fusion patterns unlock the stages of skeletal development, aiding in age estimation.

- **Sexual Dimorphism:** Explore the nuances of male and female skeletons. Features like the pelvic shape and mandible angles provide gender insights.

- **Ancestral Markers:** Navigate genetic imprints on bones. Cranial features, from nasal shapes to eye orbits, hint at ancestral roots.

- **Pathological Signatures:** Detect life's battles etched in bones. Diseases, traumas, and stress leave their imprints, contributing to the forensic narrative.

In the realm of bone identification, each fragment unfolds a story, and forensic anthropologists are the storytellers.

14.2 Age Estimation

Unlock the age secrets embedded in bones with precision:

- **Epiphyseal Fusion:** Picture the fusion dance of epiphyses. As bones mature, epiphyses unite, revealing the age tale through patterns in the long bones.

- **Dental Development:** Delve into the dental timeline. Tooth eruption, root formation, and wear patterns sculpt a roadmap for age assessment.

- **Cranial Sutures:** Examine the seams of the skull. Suture closure patterns, from sagittal to lambdoid, act as age milestones.

- **Pubic Symphysis:** Navigate the changes in the pelvic arena. Morphological shifts in the pubic symphysis reflect the aging process.

- **Auricular Surface:** Decode age nuances in the hip bone. The auricular surface, transformed by age-related changes, contributes to accuracy.

- **Sternal Rib End:** Uncover age imprints on ribs. The sternal rib end, undergoing metamorphosis, aids in fine-tuning age estimation.

In the realm of age estimation, the language of bones whispers the passage of time, allowing forensic anthropologists to decipher the age narrative.

14.3 Sex Determination

Deciphering the gender code in bones with precision:

- **Pelvic Morphology:** Visualize the pelvic puzzle. Differences in pelvic shape and size, such as the wider subpubic angle in females, offer clues to sex.

- **Sacrum Structure:** Explore sacral secrets. The broader and shorter sacrum in females contrasts with the narrower and longer sacrum in males, aiding in sex determination.

- **Skull Features:** Analyze cranial characteristics. Male skulls tend to exhibit more prominent brow ridges and larger mastoid processes compared to females.

- **Dental Traits:** Investigate dental dimorphism. Variations in tooth size, shape, and wear patterns contribute to sex determination, with males typically showing larger teeth.

- **Long Bone Dimensions:** Measure up the long bones. Differences in bone length and robusticity provide additional evidence for distinguishing between male and female skeletons.

- **Genetic Analysis:** Unlock the genetic blueprint. When skeletal features are inconclusive, DNA analysis can provide a definitive answer to sex determination.

In the quest to uncover identity from bones, forensic anthropologists harness the subtle clues embedded in skeletal remains to unravel the mystery of sex.

14.4   Stature Estimation

Unveiling height from skeletal remains with mathematical precision:

- **Long Bone Lengths:** Measure the length, unveil the height. By examining femur, tibia, and humerus lengths, forensic anthropologists employ regression equations to estimate stature.

- **Segmented Approach:** Piece by piece, estimate height. Forensic experts use formulas considering different body segments, ensuring accuracy in stature predictions.

- **Population-Specific Formulas:** Tailor-fitted precision. Formulas are often population-specific, considering variations in different ethnic groups for more accurate estimations.

- **Statistical Tools:** Crunching numbers for precision. Statistical methods refine stature estimations, providing a range of probable heights based on skeletal measurements.

- **Multivariate Analyses:** Embrace complexity for accuracy. Incorporating multiple skeletal dimensions, multivariate analyses enhance the reliability of stature estimates.

- **Molecular Insights:** Dive into the genetic pool. While skeletal measurements dominate, advancements may integrate genetic factors for a comprehensive stature estimation.

In the realm of forensic anthropology, estimating stature becomes a mathematical journey, unraveling the height of the past from bone fragments.

14.5 Trauma Analysis

Unveiling the tales hidden in bone fractures:

- **Fracture Patterns:** Decoding the language of bones. Differentiate between linear, oblique, and transverse fractures, each telling a unique story of trauma.

- **Impact Force Estimation:** From fractures to forces. Forensic anthropologists employ biomechanical principles and formulas to estimate the force applied, unveiling the intensity of the trauma.

- **Periosteal Reaction:** Bones' response to injury. Analyze periosteal reactions, where bone tissue forms in response to trauma, providing insights into the timing and nature of the event.

- **Historical Trauma:** Time-traveling through fractures. Differentiate between fresh and healed fractures, creating a timeline of traumatic events in forensic analyses.

- **Cranial Trauma Analysis:** The silent witness of head injuries. Investigate cranial fractures and their patterns, using them as clues in reconstructing the dynamics of past incidents.

- **Molecular Clues:** Delving into the chemistry of trauma. Molecular markers may provide additional insights, enhancing the understanding of bone response to injuries.

In the realm of forensic anthropology, trauma analysis unfolds the narratives written in fractures, providing a glimpse into the events of the past.

14.6 Dental Identification

Unraveling mysteries through dental clues:

- **Odontogram:** A dental fingerprint. Documenting the unique arrangement of teeth using an odontogram, aiding in identification.

- **Dental Formulas:** Deciphering the code of dentition. Utilizing dental formulas to categorize and identify individuals based on the number and types of teeth present.

- **Palatal Rugae Analysis:** The palate's secret patterns. Examining palatal rugae, the ridges in the roof of the mouth, for additional individualization in dental identification.

- **Age Estimation from Teeth:** Unveiling the age imprints. Applying age estimation formulas to dental features, providing insights into the individual's age at the time of death.

- **Dental DNA Analysis:** Molecular signatures in dental pulp. Exploring the potential of dental pulp DNA for identification, adding a genetic layer to the dental profile.

- **Chemical Composition:** Elements in enamel speak volumes. Analyzing the chemical composition of dental enamel, offering clues about the individual's geographic origin or dietary habits.

In forensic anthropology, dental identification emerges as a powerful tool, revealing a unique dental narrative.

14.7   Forensic Archaeology

Unearthing the past to solve mysteries:

- **Stratigraphy:** Layers that tell a story. Examining soil layers to understand the chronological sequence of events, aiding in crime scene reconstruction.

- **Grid Excavation:** Precision in uncovering clues. Employing grid excavation methods to systematically retrieve artifacts and remains, preserving spatial relationships.

- **Taphonomy:** Nature's impact on remains. Investigating the processes of decay, preservation, and modification of organic remains to reconstruct the post-mortem history.

- **Dating Techniques:** Timelines from the soil. Applying dating methods such as radiocarbon dating or luminescence dating to determine the age of discovered remains.

- **Artifact Analysis:** Cultural echoes in artifacts. Studying human-made objects found at a site to gain insights into the cultural practices and activities of the past.

- **GIS Mapping:** Mapping the forensic landscape. Utilizing Geographic Information System (GIS) technology to create detailed maps, aiding in spatial analysis.

In forensic anthropology, forensic archaeology serves as the time-traveling detective, revealing the secrets buried in the earth.

14.8 Mass Disasters

Navigating the aftermath of mass tragedies:

- **Humanitarian Forensic Efforts:** Uniting science and compassion. Mobilizing forensic teams to provide identifications, bringing closure to families affected by disasters.

- **Victim Recovery Protocols:** Systematic approaches in chaos. Establishing efficient protocols for the recovery of human remains, ensuring dignity and respect.

- **Ante-mortem Data Compilation:** Reconstructing identities from fragments. Compiling and comparing pre-mortem data, such as dental records and DNA profiles, to facilitate identifications.

- **Interdisciplinary Collaboration:** Strength in unity. Collaborating with diverse experts, including geneticists, odontologists, and anthropologists, to enhance identification processes.

- **Logistical Challenges:** Overcoming obstacles in the field. Addressing logistical challenges, from site accessibility to environmental conditions, to optimize recovery efforts.

- **DNA Analysis Strategies:** Decoding genetic information. Implementing advanced DNA analysis strategies, like next-generation sequencing, to enhance accuracy in victim identifications.

In the face of mass disasters, forensic anthropology emerges as a beacon of hope, piecing together the stories of those lost.

Chapter 15

Forensic Odontology

15.1 Dental Anatomy

Unveiling the intricacies of dental structures:

- **Tooth Morphology:** Unlocking the language of teeth. Explore the diverse forms and functions, from incisors to molars, shaping dental anatomy.

- **Crown and Root Features:** Deciphering the dental code. Delve into the unique features of crowns and roots, each telling a distinctive story.

- **Dental Formulas:** Formulaic revelations. Utilizing dental formulas like the Palmer notation system to describe the arrangement of teeth in human jaws.

- **Dental Occlusion:** Where form meets function. Understanding the alignment of upper and lower teeth, crucial for forensic investigations.

- **Forensic Significance:** Beyond aesthetics. Grasping the forensic importance of dental anatomy in human identification and bite mark analysis.

- **Calcium Hydroxyapatite Equation:** Molecular insights. Considering the chemical equation for calcium hydroxyapatite, the primary component of tooth enamel:

$$Ca_5(PO_4)_3(OH)$$

In the realm of forensic odontology, dental anatomy becomes a powerful tool, unraveling the mysteries within the oral landscape.

15.2   Bite Mark Analysis

Unveiling the secrets hidden in bite marks:

- **Bite Mark Characteristics:** Decoding the imprints. Explore the unique features of bite marks, such as arches, abrasions, and contusions, creating a distinctive forensic signature.

- **Human Dentition Patterns:** The dental fingerprint. Understanding how human dentition patterns, including tooth size and arrangement, imprint distinct marks on various surfaces.

- **Bite Mark Measurement Techniques:** Precision in analysis. Utilizing advanced techniques to measure and document bite marks accurately, aiding in forensic investigations.

- **Computer-Aided Bite Mark Analysis:** Bridging technology and forensics. Incorporating computational tools for enhanced precision in bite mark analysis and pattern recognition.

- **Saliva DNA Analysis:** Molecular clues in bite marks. Exploring the genetic information embedded in saliva, a potential source for DNA analysis:

$$DNA_{saliva} \rightarrow \text{Forensic Insights}$$

In the realm of forensic odontology, bite mark analysis becomes a sophisticated art, revealing stories imprinted in the most unexpected places.

15.3   Dental Records and Identification

Navigating the dental maze for forensic clarity:

- **Dental Charting:** Mapping the uniqueness. Utilizing dental charts to record individual characteristics, creating a dental profile for accurate identification.

- **Tooth Numbering Systems:** Deciphering the dental code. Understanding tooth numbering systems, such as the Palmer and FDI notation, to interpret dental records effectively.

- **Dental Radiography:** Illuminating hidden details. Harnessing the power of X-rays for comprehensive dental imaging, revealing structural nuances crucial for identification.

- **Dental Impressions:** Capturing the essence. Employing dental impressions and molds to recreate dental features, aiding in the matching process.

- **Forensic Odontogram:** The forensic blueprint. Constructing a forensic odontogram, a visual representation of dental information, streamlining the identification process.

- **DNA Analysis from Dental Samples:** Molecular echoes in dentin. Extracting DNA from dental samples for forensic genetic analysis:

$$DNA_{dental} \rightarrow \text{Identification Clues}$$

In the realm of forensic odontology, dental records emerge as a powerful tool, unlocking the gates to precise identification.

15.4 Age Estimation from Teeth

Deciphering the age code embedded in dental structures:

- **Dental Development:** Unraveling the growth narrative. Examining tooth eruption patterns and stages of dental development as a timeline to estimate age.

- **Dental Wear Analysis:** Tracing the footsteps of time. Analyzing dental wear, considering factors like attrition and abrasion, to gauge the wear-and-tear journey of teeth.

- **Root Dentin Transparency:** A translucent window to the past. Measuring root dentin transparency as an indicator of age progression, offering a glimpse into the history of the tooth.

- **Cementum Analysis:** Counting the rings of dentition. Assessing cementum layers to determine age, akin to counting rings in a tree trunk, revealing the annual growth story.

- **Age Estimation Formulas:** Mathematizing the age puzzle. Employing age estimation formulas, such as $Formula_1$ and $Formula_2$, incorporating tooth dimensions and developmental stages:

$$\text{Age}_{\text{estimated}} = \text{Formula}_1 + \text{Formula}_2$$

- **Molecular Age Markers:** Delving into molecular timekeeping. Exploring molecular age markers within dental tissues, unlocking age-related genetic information:

$$\text{Molecular}_{\text{age}} \rightarrow \text{Age}_{\text{Estimation}}$$

In the intricate world of forensic odontology, teeth hold the key to unraveling the enigma of age.

15.5   Dental Evidence in Abuse Cases

Unraveling the silent testimony of teeth in cases of abuse:

- **Patterns of Dental Injuries:** Decoding the language of trauma. Analyzing dental injuries, including fractures and patterns of trauma, to construct a narrative of potential abuse.

- **Age Assessment in Abuse Cases:** Merging age estimation with abuse investigations. Utilizing age estimation techniques, such as $\text{Formula}_{\text{Age}}$, to determine if the observed injuries align with the victim's age.

- **Bite Mark Analysis:** Teeth as unique fingerprints. Examining bite marks, applying forensic techniques like $\text{Analysis}_{\text{BiteMark}}$, to link dental evidence to potential perpetrators.

- **Dental Records and Documentation:** The paper trail within the mouth. Scrutinizing dental records, employing $\text{Documentation}_{\text{Forensic}}$, to establish a comprehensive history and timeline of oral health.

- **Chemical Analysis of Dental Materials:** Tracing origins through composition. Conducting chemical analysis, utilizing $\text{Analytical}_{\text{Chemistry}}$, to identify dental materials, potentially connecting the victim to a specific location.

- **Molecular Evidence:** DNA whispers within dental tissues. Extracting molecular evidence, using $\text{DNA}_{\text{Extraction}}$ techniques, to unveil genetic markers that might link the victim to an abuser.

- **Tooth Mark Analysis on Objects:** Connecting the dots through tooth marks. Investigating tooth marks on objects with $Analysis_{ToothMark}$, aiming to link dental evidence to potential crime scenes.

- **Psychological Evaluation:** Beyond physical signs. Integrating psychological evaluations, employing $Psychological_{Evaluation}$, to comprehend the impact of dental abuse on the victim.

In the realm of forensic odontology, teeth emerge not only as witnesses but also as storytellers in cases of abuse.

15.6 Forensic Photography

Capturing the essence of forensic odontology through the lens:

- **Photographic Documentation:** Freeze-framing dental evidence. Employing $Documentation_{Photographic}$ techniques to capture high-quality images of dental features for analysis.

- **Scale and Calibration:** Precision in pixels. Utilizing $Calibration_{Photographic}$ methods to ensure accurate measurements of dental characteristics in forensic images.

- **Lighting Techniques:** Illuminating the details. Applying $Lighting_{Forensic}$ strategies to enhance visibility and reveal intricate features in dental photographs.

- **Macro Photography:** Zooming into the microcosm. Utilizing $Photography_{Macro}$ to capture minute details of dental evidence, aiding in comprehensive analysis.

- **UV and Infrared Photography:** Beyond the visible spectrum. Leveraging $Photography_{UV/Infrared}$ to unveil hidden details in dental evidence not perceivable under standard lighting.

- **Three-Dimensional Imaging:** Adding depth to analysis. Implementing $Imaging_{3D}$ techniques for a more holistic view of dental features, facilitating thorough examination.

- **Image Enhancement Tools:** Unveiling the hidden. Using $Enhancement_{Tools}$ to sharpen, clarify, and reveal obscured details in dental photographs.

- **Forensic Video Analysis:** Dynamic storytelling. Integrating $Video_{Forensic}$ for a real-time depiction of dental evidence, aiding in dynamic analysis.

- **Ethical Considerations:** Respecting the visual narrative. Adhering to Ethical$_{\text{Photography}}$ standards to ensure the respectful and responsible capture of forensic odontological evidence.

In forensic odontology, every photograph is a visual testament, unraveling the mysteries held within dental evidence.

15.7   Digital Imaging in Forensics

Navigating the pixels of forensic odontology with digital precision:

- **Digital Radiography:** Transcending traditional X-rays. Harnessing Radiography$_{\text{Digital}}$ for high-resolution dental images, aiding in detailed forensic analysis.

- **Intraoral Scanning:** Beyond the surface. Employing Scanning$_{\text{Intraoral}}$ technologies to capture intricate dental details in three dimensions for comprehensive examination.

- **3D Reconstruction:** Building dental landscapes. Utilizing Reconstruction$_{\text{3D}}$ techniques to assemble a virtual representation of dental features, facilitating in-depth analysis.

- **Computer-Aided Design (CAD):** From pixels to precision. Integrating Design$_{\text{CAD}}$ tools to enhance accuracy in the creation and examination of dental prosthetics and reconstructions.

- **Comparison Software:** Pixels meet patterns. Leveraging Software$_{\text{Comparison}}$ for side-by-side analysis of dental images, streamlining the identification process.

- **Biometrics in Forensic Dentistry:** Uniqueness in dentition. Applying Biometrics$_{\text{Dental}}$ for individual identification based on distinct dental features, enhancing forensic accuracy.

- **Data Encryption and Security:** Safeguarding the digital archive. Implementing Encryption$_{\text{Data}}$ to protect sensitive dental records, ensuring the integrity of forensic data.

- **Virtual Autopsy:** Navigating the digital cadaver. Embracing Autopsy$_{\text{Virtual}}$ for a detailed examination of dental structures in a virtual forensic environment.

- **Integration with Forensic Databases:** Connecting the dots. Linking digital dental records with Forensic$_{\text{Databases}}$ for efficient cross-referencing and identification.

In the realm of forensic odontology, pixels become forensic storytellers, revealing the intricate details of dental evidence through digital imaging.

15.8 Legal Issues in Forensic Odontology

Navigating the legal landscape of dental evidence with precision:

- **Admissibility of Dental Evidence:** From court to canines. Ensuring the $Evidence_{Dental}$ meets legal standards for admissibility, establishing its reliability in forensic proceedings.

- **Expert Witness Testimony:** Words as evidence. Crafting $Testimony_{Expert}$ that effectively communicates dental findings to the court, establishing credibility and aiding in legal decision-making.

- **Chain of Custody:** Preserving the dental trail. Implementing $Custody_{Chain}$ protocols to document the handling of dental evidence, maintaining its integrity and reliability in legal proceedings.

- **Forensic Odontologist as Consultant:** A dental guide in the legal maze. Serving as a $Consultant_{Forensic\ Odontologist}$ to legal professionals, offering insights into dental evidence interpretation and significance.

- **Ethical Considerations:** Navigating the moral compass. Adhering to $Considerations_{Ethical}$ in the collection, analysis, and presentation of dental evidence, upholding professional integrity in legal contexts.

- **Legal Standards for Bite Mark Analysis:** Defining dental imprints. Establishing $Standards_{Legal}$ for the analysis and interpretation of $Bite\ Marks_{Dental}$, ensuring accuracy and reliability in legal proceedings.

- **Role of Forensic Odontologist in Legal Investigations:** Beyond the dental chair. Defining the $Role_{Forensic\ Odontologist}$ in legal investigations, clarifying responsibilities and contributions to legal outcomes.

- **Privacy and Confidentiality:** Guarding dental secrets. Upholding $Privacy_{Dental}$ and $Confidentiality_{Forensic}$ in the handling of dental records, respecting the rights of individuals and maintaining professional standards.

In the realm of legal considerations, forensic odontology stands as a sentinel, ensuring the lawful integration of dental evidence in the pursuit of justice.

Chapter 16

Forensic Pathology

16.1 Overview

Unveiling the secrets of the deceased with forensic precision:

- **Postmortem Examination:** The Examination$_{\text{Postmortem}}$ ritual begins, a meticulous exploration of the deceased's remains, unraveling the mysteries concealed within.

- **Cause of Death Determination:** Decoding the Cause$_{\text{Death}}$ puzzle. Employing medical expertise and investigative tools to pinpoint the catalyst that led to the cessation of life.

- **Time Since Death Estimation:** A journey through Time$_{\text{Since Death}}$. Utilizing scientific methods, from rigor mortis to forensic entomology, to decipher the temporal aspects of mortality.

- **Manner of Death Classification:** Sorting the Manner$_{\text{Death}}$ mosaic. Distinguishing between natural, accidental, suicidal, homicidal, or undetermined paths that led to the ultimate fate.

- **Forensic Autopsy Techniques:** The artistry of Autopsy$_{\text{Forensic}}$. Applying surgical precision to extract information, unveiling the narrative inscribed within the anatomy of the deceased.

- **Toxicology Analysis:** Unmasking Toxicology$_{\text{Analysis}}$. Delving into bodily fluids and tissues to identify the presence of toxins, drugs, or poisons that might have contributed to the demise.

- **Forensic Anthropology in Identification:** The skeletal whispers. Integrating

Anthropology$_{\text{Forensic}}$ to establish the identity of the departed, a crucial step in the forensic puzzle.

- **Documentation and Report Crafting:** The Documentation$_{\text{Forensic}}$ saga unfolds. Translating findings into comprehensive reports, a cornerstone in conveying forensic insights to legal entities.

In the realm of forensic pathology, each examination unveils a chapter in the untold story, contributing to the pursuit of truth and justice.

16.2   Mechanism of Death

Exploring the intricate machinery that orchestrates life's final curtain call:

- **Cardiopulmonary Failure ($CP_{\textbf{Failure}}$):** Witness the cessation of the Cardiopulmonary$_{\text{System}}$ symphony. When the heart and lungs cease their harmonious rhythm, life succumbs to their silence.

- **Hypovolemic Shock ($HS_{\textbf{Shock}}$):** The Hypovolemic$_{\text{Drama}}$ unfolds. With a dramatic loss of blood volume, the body's vital organs starve for nourishment, triggering a cascade towards mortality.

- **Neurological Dysfunction ($ND_{\textbf{Dysfunction}}$):** Delve into the enigma of Neurological$_{\text{Chaos}}$. When the brain's intricate dance falters, consciousness wanes, leading to the final curtain in the theater of life.

- **Respiratory Arrest ($RA_{\textbf{Arrest}}$):** Witness the Respiratory$_{\text{Curtain}}$ descent. As breath, the essence of life, falters and fades, the body succumbs to the quietude of respiratory arrest.

- **Multi-Organ Failure ($MOF_{\textbf{Failure}}$):** The tragic Multi-Organ$_{\text{Tragedy}}$ unfolds. When organs engage in a sorrowful symphony of failure, the body's resilience crumbles, succumbing to the inevitable.

- **Metabolic Derangement ($MD_{\textbf{Derangement}}$):** Unravel the metabolic Metabolic$_{\text{Turbulence}}$. When the body's chemical orchestra loses its harmony, a cascade of derangement ensues, leading to life's dissolution.

In the theater of forensic pathology, understanding the $Mechanism_{\text{Death}}$ illuminates the intricate choreography that concludes life's performance.

16.3   Wound Analysis

Unveiling the silent narratives etched in wounds, where every mark tells a story:

- **Blunt Force Trauma (BFT_{Trauma}):** Navigate the aftermath of $Blunt_{\text{Force}}$ encounters. Energy dissipates through tissues, leaving a trail of contusions, fractures, and the silent testimony of impact.

- **Sharp Force Injuries (SFI_{Injuries}):** Witness the precision of $Sharp_{\text{Force}}$. Blades, puncturing with intent, carve tales in flesh. Stab wounds and incisions whisper of encounters with edged instruments.

- **Firearm-related Injuries (FRI_{Injuries}):** Unravel the ballistic narratives scripted by $Firearm_{\text{Ballet}}$. Gunshot wounds, with their unique signatures, echo the deadly ballet between projectiles and flesh.

- **Asphyxial Injuries (AI_{Injuries}):** Peer into the world of breathless struggles with $Asphyxial_{\text{Encounters}}$. Strangulation, suffocation, and drowning leave their imprints on the canvas of the deceased.

- **Thermal Injuries (TI_{Injuries}):** Feel the burn of $Thermal_{\text{Chaos}}$. Flames and scalds inscribe tales of fiery encounters, leaving behind the scars of thermal trauma.

- **Chemical and Toxicological Injuries (CTI_{Injuries}):** Navigate the toxic terrain of $Chemical_{\text{Encounters}}$. Poisons and toxins, silent assassins, script their stories within the body's internal landscape.

In the realm of forensic pathology, decoding wounds reveals the untold sagas of life's violent chapters.

16.4   Asphyxia and Strangulation

Unraveling the silent narratives of breathless encounters:

- **Asphyxia** ($A_{\mathbf{Asphyxia}}$): Dive into the suffocating embrace of Asphyxia, where the oxygen supply is disrupted. Struggle for breath, a silent plea etched in the stillness.

- **Strangulation** ($S_{\mathbf{Strangulation}}$): Feel the grip of Strangulation as external forces tighten around the neck. Marks of violence, a macabre ballet between the assailant and the breathless victim.

- **Hanging** ($H_{\mathbf{Hanging}}$): Explore the complexities of Hanging, where the body succumbs to gravity's cruel dance. Marks of suspension, a deadly performance scripted by the laws of physics.

- **Choking** ($C_{\mathbf{Choking}}$): Witness the desperate struggle in Choking, where foreign bodies obstruct the airway. Gasps for air, a silent battle against the obstruction within.

- **Smothering** ($S_{\mathbf{Smothering}}$): Enter the realm of Smothering, where external forces stifle the breath. The absence of air, a sinister tale of breath denied.

- **Positional Asphyxia** ($PA_{\mathbf{Asphyxia}}$): Understand the lethal dance of Positional$_{\mathrm{Asphyxia}}$, where body positioning becomes a fatal factor. The silent compromise of physiological balance.

In the realm of forensic pathology, Asphyxia and Strangulation whisper tales of breath stolen and lives extinguished.

16.5   Blunt Force Injuries

Unravel the secrets of blunt force trauma with simplified insights:

- **Kinetic Energy (KE):**

$$KE = \frac{1}{2}mv^2$$

Where m is mass and v is velocity.

- **Types of Blunt Force Injuries:**

  1. **Contusion:** Think of it as a bruise, caused by blunt impact without breaking the skin.

  2. **Abrasion:** Visualize superficial damage, like a scrape on the skin due to friction.

  3. **Laceration:** Imagine deeper cuts, involving tearing of tissues.

- **Fracture Patterns:**

  - **Linear Fractures:** Straight-line breaks often seen in flat bones.

  - **Comminuted Fractures:** Splintering into multiple fragments, common in high-velocity impacts.

- **Trauma Analysis:**

  - **Trajectory Reconstruction:** Trace the path of the impacting force to understand the dynamics.

  - **Injury Severity:** Consider kinetic energy, impact surface, and victim's anatomy.

- **Molecular Insight:**

  - **Calcium Signaling:** Highlighting cellular responses to mechanical stress.

  - **Collagen Disruption:** Understanding structural damage at the molecular level.

Blunt force injuries tell a story – decoding these signs is key to reconstructing events and unveiling the truth.

16.6   Sharp Force Injuries

Explore the world of sharp force injuries with simplicity:

- **Force and Penetration:**

$$P = F/A$$

  where P is pressure, F is force, and A is the area.

- **Types of Sharp Force Injuries:**

  1. **Incised Wound:** Visualize a clean, smooth cut, often deeper than it is wide.

  2. **Stab Wound:** Envision a deeper, narrow wound, often caused by a pointed weapon.

  3. **Chop Wound:** Imagine a heavy, hacking blow causing a distinctive injury pattern.

- **Wound Analysis:**

  - **Directionality:** Examine the orientation of the wound to understand the weapon's path.

- **Wound Healing:** Consider the body's response, aiding in timeline estimation.

- **Molecular Insights:**

  - **Hemostasis Cascade:** Delve into the body's intricate blood clotting response.

  - **Tissue Repair:** Explore the molecular mechanisms orchestrating wound healing.

Sharp force injuries leave distinct marks – decoding them is like unraveling a forensic puzzle.

16.7   Gunshot Wounds

Unveil the mysteries of gunshot wounds with simplicity:

- **Ballistics Basics:** Picture bullets in motion and the science of their trajectory.

- **Wound Ballistics:** Imagine the dynamic interaction between bullets and tissues.

- **Firearm Types:** Recognize handguns, rifles, and shotguns – each leaving a unique imprint.

- **Gunshot Residue Analysis:** Explore the aftermath, detecting firearm discharge residues.

- **Internal Ballistics:** Envision the bullet's journey within the barrel before it sets its course.

- **External Ballistics:** Understand factors influencing the bullet's flight path after leaving the barrel.

- **Terminal Ballistics:** Explore the bullet's impact and interaction with tissues upon contact.

- **Molecular Insights:** Dive into the forensic analysis of gunshot residue and its chemical signatures.

Gunshot wounds tell a tale written in ballistic patterns and tissue reactions.

16.8   Forensic Entomology

Embark on the fascinating journey of insects in forensic investigations:

- **Insect Arrival Patterns:** Picture the systematic timeline of insects colonizing a cadaver.

- **Maggot Development:** Understand the life cycles of maggots, key players in postmortem intervals.

- **Entomological Succession:** Envision the changing cast of insect characters and their chronological appearance.

- **Temperature's Role:** Explore how ambient temperature influences insect activity and decomposition rates.

- **Entomotoxicology:** Delve into the study of toxins in insects, providing clues to the cause of death.

- **Forensic Acarology:** Recognize the role of mites and ticks in forensic entomology.

- **Applications in Legal Cases:** See how insect evidence becomes a crucial witness in courtrooms.

- **Collection and Preservation:** Learn the art of gathering and conserving entomological evidence.

Insects, the silent investigators of time, reveal the secrets of postmortem timelines.

Chapter 17

Forensic Toxicology

17.1 Introduction to Toxicology

Dive into the world of toxins and their forensic implications:

- **Toxic Substances:** Explore a myriad of substances that can cause harm to the human body.

- **Dose-Response Relationship:** Understand the correlation between the dose of a substance and its effects.

- **Routes of Exposure:** Navigate the various pathways through which toxins enter the body.

- **Absorption and Distribution:** Witness the journey of toxins within the body, from entry to systemic circulation.

- **Metabolism and Elimination:** Uncover the body's mechanisms for processing and expelling toxic compounds.

- **Toxicological Analysis Methods:** Explore techniques like chromatography and mass spectrometry for detecting toxins.

- **Toxicokinetics:** Envision the study of how the body interacts with and responds to toxic substances over time.

- **Case Studies:** Delve into real-world examples showcasing the role of toxicology in solving crimes.

Toxicology, the silent investigator of poisons, decodes the mysteries of harmful substances.

17.2   Classes of Poisons

Embark on a journey through the diverse realms of poisons:

- **Heavy Metals:** Encounter the toxic allure of metals like lead, mercury, and arsenic, disrupting physiological processes.

- **Alkaloids:** Explore the world of plant-derived poisons, from the deadly nightshade to the intriguing effects of caffeine.

- **Gases:** Enter the invisible realm of toxic gases, where substances like carbon monoxide and hydrogen cyanide pose lethal threats.

- **Narcotics:** Navigate the landscape of opioids and other narcotics, understanding their pain-relieving and toxic effects.

- **Volatile Substances:** Inhale the dangers of volatile compounds, from solvents to household chemicals, impacting the nervous system.

- **Pesticides and Herbicides:** Witness the agricultural poisons designed to eliminate pests, with potential harm to humans.

- **Toxic Plants:** Explore the botanical world of poisonous plants, where innocuous-looking flora can conceal deadly toxins.

- **Chemical Warfare Agents:** Uncover the sinister side of chemical warfare, where agents like sarin and mustard gas wreak havoc on the human body.

In the realm of forensic toxicology, understanding poison classes is the key to unraveling mysterious deaths.

17.3   Methods of Toxicological Analysis

Embark on the analytical odyssey of forensic toxicology:

- **Chromatography:** Peer into the separation magic of chromatography, where toxins reveal themselves through distinct patterns.

- **Mass Spectrometry:** Dive into the molecular realm with mass spectrometry, identifying toxins by their unique mass-to-charge ratios.

- **Immunoassays:** Unlock the power of antibodies in immunoassays, detecting toxins through specific antigen-antibody interactions.

- **Spectrophotometry:** Witness the play of light in spectrophotometry, measuring toxin concentrations based on their absorption or emission.

- **Enzyme-linked Immunosorbent Assay (ELISA):** Delve into ELISA, a versatile tool using enzymes to signal the presence of toxins.

- **Polymerase Chain Reaction (PCR):** Enter the genetic realm with PCR, amplifying DNA for precise identification of toxin-related genes.

- **Nuclear Magnetic Resonance (NMR):** Explore the magnetic signatures in NMR, unraveling toxin structures with atomic precision.

- **X-Ray Crystallography:** Peer into the crystal lattice with X-ray crystallography, visualizing toxin molecules in intricate detail.

In the forensic laboratory, these methods illuminate the shadowy presence of toxins, guiding investigators to the truth.

17.4   Drug Metabolism

Embark on the metabolic journey of drugs:

- **Phase I Metabolism:** Witness the transformation in Phase I, where drugs undergo oxidation, reduction, or hydrolysis, often catalyzed by cytochrome P450 enzymes.

- **Phase II Metabolism:** Experience the conjugation phase, where drug metabolites combine with endogenous substances (glucuronic acid, sulfate, etc.), enhancing water solubility.

- **Enzymatic Reactions:** Dive into the enzymatic ballet as drug molecules interact with metabolic enzymes, evolving into more polar and easily excretable forms.

- **Liver's Central Role:** Envision the liver as the metabolic maestro, orchestrating drug biotransformation with precision.

- **Prodrugs Unveiled:** Explore the strategy of prodrugs, inert compounds that transform into active drugs upon metabolism, optimizing therapeutic effects.

- **Metabolism and Drug Testing:** Grasp the significance in drug testing, where metabolites serve as fingerprints, revealing recent drug exposure.

- **Individual Variation:** Acknowledge the diversity in drug metabolism among individuals, influencing drug response and toxicity.

- **Pharmacogenomics:** Navigate the genomic landscape, understanding how genetic variations impact drug metabolism and individualized treatment.

In the intricate dance of drug metabolism, the body choreographs a symphony of transformations, shaping the fate of pharmaceutical agents.

17.5   Postmortem Redistribution

Unveil the mysteries of postmortem drug redistribution:

- **Postmortem Changes:** Witness the dynamic alterations in drug distribution postmortem, impacting concentrations in various tissues.

- **Factors Influencing Redistribution:** Explore the variables shaping postmortem drug movement, including tissue permeability, blood pooling, and decomposition.

- **Drug Redistribution Models:** Dive into mathematical models capturing the intricate dynamics of postmortem drug redistribution, aiding forensic interpretations.

- **Significance in Toxicology:** Grasp the implications for toxicological analyses, as postmortem redistribution may confound accurate determination of antemortem drug levels.

- **Analytical Challenges:** Navigate the challenges faced by forensic toxicologists in distinguishing between postmortem changes and actual drug exposure.

- **Interpretation Nuances:** Understand the nuanced interpretation required in cases involving postmortem redistribution, balancing scientific rigor with real-world complexity.

- **Prevention Strategies:** Envision strategies to mitigate postmortem redistribution effects, enhancing the accuracy of toxicological findings.

- **Advancements in Analysis:** Explore evolving techniques and technologies aiming to refine the understanding and mitigation of postmortem drug redistribution.

In the realm of forensic toxicology, unraveling the intricacies of postmortem redistribution adds a layer of complexity to the interpretation of drug concentrations.

17.6 Toxicological Interpretation

Decode the language of toxicology for a comprehensive interpretation:

- **Dose-Response Relationships:** Uncover the correlation between the dose of a substance and its observed effects, a fundamental principle in toxicological interpretation.

- **Threshold Levels:** Explore the concept of threshold levels, the point below which a substance poses minimal risk, providing key insights into safety margins.

- **Acute vs. Chronic Exposure:** Differentiate between acute and chronic exposure scenarios, recognizing the varied effects on the body over different timeframes.

- **Metabolism and Biotransformation:** Delve into the metabolic fate of toxicants, understanding how the body transforms substances and the implications for toxicity.

- **Bioavailability and Absorption:** Grasp the significance of bioavailability and absorption rates in determining the actual dose reaching target organs.

- **Interindividual Variability:** Navigate the complexities of individual differences in response to toxicants, considering genetic, physiological, and lifestyle factors.

- **Synergistic and Antagonistic Effects:** Explore the interactive effects of substances, whether amplifying (synergistic) or diminishing (antagonistic) each other's impact.

- **Forensic Implications:** Apply toxicological principles to forensic scenarios, discerning between therapeutic, toxic, and lethal levels for a precise interpretation.

In the realm of forensic toxicology, a nuanced understanding of toxicological interpretation is the key to unraveling the mysteries hidden within toxicological reports.

17.7   Case Studies

Embark on forensic journeys through real-world cases, unraveling toxicological mysteries:

- **The Cyanide Conundrum:** Investigate a case involving cyanide poisoning, examining the dose-response relationship and identifying the source through meticulous analysis.

- **Over-the-Counter Overdose:** Explore the repercussions of an overdose on a common over-the-counter medication, delving into metabolism rates and factors influencing toxicity.

- **Alcohol and Accusations:** Untangle the complexities of alcohol-related cases, considering postmortem redistribution and the influence of individual variability on blood alcohol concentration.

- **Designer Drug Dilemma:** Navigate the challenges posed by designer drugs, where metabolites and evolving chemical structures present unique hurdles in toxicological interpretation.

- **Environmental Exposures:** Investigate cases involving environmental toxicants, highlighting the importance of absorption, bioavailability, and the interplay with chronic exposure.

- **Polypharmacy Puzzle:** Decipher cases involving multiple drug interactions, analyzing synergistic and antagonistic effects to determine the cumulative impact on the body.

- **Forensic Pharmacogenomics:** Explore the intersection of genetics and toxicology, examining cases where an individual's genetic makeup influences drug response and toxicity.

- **Legal Implications:** Delve into cases with legal ramifications, where toxicological findings play a pivotal role in establishing causation, culpability, and legal consequences.

In the realm of forensic toxicology, case studies serve as windows into the intricacies of real-life scenarios, enriching our understanding of toxicological principles.

17.8   Forensic Pharmacology

Embark on a journey through the intricate world of forensic pharmacology, where drugs and their interactions weave a complex narrative:

- **Drug Dynamics:** Unravel the dynamics of drug action, exploring concepts like absorption, distribution, metabolism, and excretion (ADME), crucial in understanding a substance's journey through the body.

- **Pharmacokinetics Puzzle:** Dive into the puzzle of pharmacokinetics, deciphering equations that govern drug concentration over time, influencing dosage regimens and forensic interpretations.

- **Receptor Relationships:** Explore the intricate relationships between drugs and receptors, understanding binding kinetics and how receptor interactions mediate therapeutic effects and toxicity.

- **Enzymatic Enigma:** Investigate the role of enzymes in drug metabolism, demystifying the enzymatic transformations that impact a substance's activity and contribute to interindividual variations.

- **Toxicokinetics Tangle:** Navigate the tangle of toxicokinetics, examining how the body handles toxic substances, and the factors influencing the onset, intensity, and duration of toxic effects.

- **Interactions Interlude:** Delve into drug-drug interactions, exploring the synergies and conflicts that arise when multiple substances coexist in the body, shaping forensic outcomes.

- **Metabolic Machinery:** Explore the metabolic machinery behind drug biotransformation, visualizing enzymatic reactions and their impact on drug clearance and toxicity.

- **Forensic Formulations:** Examine the forensic formulations of pharmaceuticals, understanding how drug formulations influence absorption rates, bioavailability, and subsequent toxicological outcomes.

In the realm of forensic pharmacology, the interplay between drugs and the human body unfolds as a captivating story, each chapter revealing the secrets of substance interactions.

Chapter 18

Forensic Serology and DNA Analysis

18.1 Blood and Bloodstains

Embark on a forensic journey into the realm of blood and bloodstains, where each droplet tells a story:

- **Blood Components:** Unveil the secrets held within blood components—plasma, red blood cells, white blood cells, and platelets—each playing a unique role in forensic investigations.

- **Serological Sleuthing:** Explore the art of serological analysis, deciphering blood types using ABO and Rh systems, creating a roadmap for identifying individuals and excluding potential contributors.

- **Presumptive Tests:** Dive into the world of presumptive tests, employing chemical reactions to detect the presence of blood, guiding forensic investigators to potential crime scenes and crucial evidence.

- **Genetic Signatures:** Decode the genetic signatures within blood, understanding DNA profiling techniques like short tandem repeat (STR) analysis, a powerful tool for individual identification.

- **Stain Patterns:** Analyze bloodstain patterns, where the size, shape, and distribution of stains provide insights into the dynamics of a crime—whether it's a result of impact, gunshot, or arterial spray.

- **Luminol Luminescence:** Illuminate crime scenes with luminol, visualizing blood that has been cleaned or is not visible to the naked eye, revealing hidden traces critical for forensic reconstruction.

- **Coagulation Chronicles:** Explore the coagulation process, understanding how blood clotting influences the appearance of stains, contributing valuable information to forensic analyses.

- **Forensic Artistry:** Witness the forensic artistry of bloodstain pattern analysis, where skilled investigators reconstruct events based on the physics of blood in motion, shedding light on the sequence of actions.

In the world of forensic serology and DNA analysis, blood becomes a silent witness, narrating the story of a crime through its biochemical and genetic signatures.

18.2   Blood Group Systems

Embark on a genetic exploration of blood group systems, where the alphabet of blood reveals intricate details:

- **ABO System:** Unravel the ABO system, where the presence or absence of A and B antigens defines blood types—A, B, AB, and O—creating the foundation for blood compatibility and transfusions.

- **Rh System:** Navigate the Rh system, distinguishing between Rh-positive (+) and Rh-negative (-) blood types, crucial in understanding blood compatibility and preventing transfusion reactions.

- **MN System:** Delve into the MN system, where the M and N antigens contribute additional layers of complexity to blood typing, enhancing the precision of forensic investigations.

- **Lewis System:** Explore the Lewis system, unveiling the intricacies of Lewis antigens, providing supplementary information for forensic serologists to decipher blood-related mysteries.

- **Duffy System:** Journey into the Duffy system, where distinct antigens play a role in blood-cell interactions, adding nuances to the broader landscape of blood group diversity.

- **Kell System:** Enter the realm of the Kell system, where Kell antigens contribute to a comprehensive understanding of blood types, offering valuable insights in forensic serology.

- **Diego System:** Examine the Diego system, where Diego antigens become integral puzzle pieces, aiding forensic scientists in painting a detailed picture of blood characteristics.

- **Secretor Status:** Uncover the secretor status, a genetic trait influencing the presence of blood group antigens in bodily fluids, enhancing the interpretive power of forensic analyses.

In the intricate language of blood group systems, each letter and antigen tells a unique tale, empowering forensic serologists to decode the genetic information embedded in blood.

18.3   DNA Structure and Function

Embark on a microscopic journey through the elegant world of DNA, where the code of life is written in molecular poetry:

- **Double Helix Dance:** Witness the mesmerizing double helix, where DNA's two strands intertwine like partners in a molecular dance, forming the iconic structure that encodes genetic information.

- **Nucleotide Ballet:** Marvel at the nucleotide ballet, where adenine (A), thymine (T), cytosine (C), and guanine (G) pirouette in pairs, creating the genetic language that spells out the instructions for life.

- **Base Pairing Symphony:** Listen to the base pairing symphony, where A harmoniously pairs with T, and C elegantly pairs with G, composing the genetic melody that ensures fidelity in DNA replication.

- **DNA Replication Ballet:** Attend the DNA replication ballet, a choreographed spectacle where the double helix gracefully unwinds, and new strands emerge, duplicating the genetic code with precision.

- **Transcription Waltz:** Join the transcription waltz, where DNA's poetic script is transcribed into messenger RNA (mRNA), preparing the stage for protein synthesis.

- **Translation Pas de Deux:** Experience the translation pas de deux, as mRNA and transfer RNA (tRNA) collaborate to assemble amino acids, crafting proteins that orchestrate the body's functions.

- **Genetic Orchestra:** Envision the genetic orchestra, where the symphony of genes plays a unique composition for each individual, defining traits, characteristics, and the essence of life.

In the enchanting realm of DNA, the choreography of molecules unfolds the saga of life, revealing the intricate dance that shapes our existence.

18.4   Forensic DNA Typing

Delve into the fascinating world of forensic DNA typing, where the language of genes becomes a powerful tool for criminal investigations:

- **STR Profiling Ballet:** Witness the STR profiling ballet, where Short Tandem Repeats (STRs) take center stage. These repeating genetic sequences create unique patterns, like individual dancers, distinguishing one person from another.

- **Polymerase Chain Reaction (PCR) Symphony:** Listen to the PCR symphony, a molecular crescendo that amplifies tiny DNA samples, allowing forensic analysts to compose a genetic symphony from the smallest biological traces.

- **Gel Electrophoresis Performance:** Attend the gel electrophoresis performance, where DNA fragments elegantly glide through a gel matrix, creating distinct bands that form the genetic score played by each individual.

- **Capillary Electrophoresis Waltz:** Engage in the capillary electrophoresis waltz, a high-tech dance that separates DNA fragments based on size, producing a precise genetic fingerprint for identification.

- **Mitochondrial DNA Ballet:** Experience the mitochondrial DNA ballet, where the maternally inherited DNA performs a unique routine. Though slower-paced, it unveils historical connections and aids in tracing ancestry.

- **Forensic DNA Database Harmony:** Envision the forensic DNA database harmony, where genetic profiles harmonize in vast databases, helping investigators link evidence to individuals and solve mysteries.

- **Genetic Cold Case Resolution:** Marvel at the genetic cold case resolution, as advancements in DNA typing revive dormant cases, bringing justice to victims and closure to their families.

In the mesmerizing arena of forensic DNA typing, the language of genetics becomes a powerful instrument, revealing the stories hidden within our DNA.

18.5   DNA Profiling Techniques

Embark on a journey through the intricate world of DNA profiling techniques, where the code of life becomes a forensic masterpiece:

- **PCR Elegance:** Witness the elegance of Polymerase Chain Reaction (PCR), where the DNA amplification process unfolds like a molecular ballet, multiplying trace amounts of genetic material.

- **Gel Electrophoresis Symphony:** Attend the gel electrophoresis symphony, a genetic orchestra where charged DNA fragments move through a gel matrix, creating distinct patterns that form an individual's unique genetic melody.

- **Capillary Electrophoresis Waltz:** Engage in the capillary electrophoresis waltz, a high-tech dance that separates DNA fragments based on size, revealing the intricate genetic details that compose a person's identity.

- **STR Profiling Ballet:** Marvel at the STR profiling ballet, where Short Tandem Repeats (STRs) take the stage, dancing in unique patterns that differentiate one person from another in the forensic genetic score.

- **Mitochondrial DNA Saga:** Explore the mitochondrial DNA saga, a slower-paced narrative that traces maternal lineage, providing insights into ancestry and connecting individuals across generations.

- **Forensic DNA Database Ensemble:** Envision the forensic DNA database ensemble, where genetic profiles harmonize to create a vast repository, aiding investigators in solving crimes and identifying individuals.

- **Revolutionary Genetic Technologies:** Delve into the revolutionary genetic technologies shaping the future of DNA profiling, promising breakthroughs in solving cold cases and unraveling genetic mysteries.

In the realm of forensic DNA profiling, each technique contributes to a symphony of knowledge, unraveling the secrets encoded in the strands of life.

18.6 Mitochondrial DNA Analysis

Embark on a journey into the ancient DNA realm, where the power of mitochondria unveils stories hidden in the maternal lineage:

- **Mitochondrial DNA Unveiling:** Imagine the unveiling of mitochondrial DNA, a genetic time capsule passed down from mothers, holding the key to exploring ancestry and tracing familial connections.

- **PCR Amplification Symphony:** Dive into the PCR amplification symphony, where targeted regions of mitochondrial DNA undergo an elegant amplification process, creating copies for forensic scrutiny.

- **Sequencing Ballet:** Witness the sequencing ballet, a choreography of nucleotides revealing the genetic script. High-throughput sequencing technologies decipher the mitochondrial code with unprecedented precision.

- **Haplogroup Heritage Waltz:** Engage in the haplogroup heritage waltz, where the analysis of specific mitochondrial DNA variations leads to the identification of haplogroups, connecting individuals to broader ancestral populations.

- **Forensic Applications Overture:** Experience the forensic applications overture, as mitochondrial DNA analysis plays a pivotal role in scenarios where nuclear DNA may be scarce or degraded, offering a reliable investigative tool.

- **Maternal Lineage Opera:** Delve into the maternal lineage opera, where mitochondrial DNA becomes a storyteller, narrating the journey of generations and providing valuable insights for forensic investigators.

- **Advancements and Challenges Duet:** Explore the advancements and challenges duet, as mitochondrial DNA analysis evolves with technological strides, presenting new opportunities and complexities in the forensic landscape.

In the world of mitochondrial DNA analysis, every sequence echoes the footsteps of ancestors, guiding forensic investigators through the intricate tapestry of genetic history.

18.7 Challenges in DNA Analysis

Embark on the journey of unraveling the complexities woven into the strands of DNA analysis, where challenges spark innovation and resilience:

- **Degraded DNA Puzzle:** Imagine the challenge of piecing together a degraded DNA puzzle. In forensic scenarios, where DNA may be fragmented or compromised, cutting-edge techniques like low-template DNA analysis strive to reconstruct the genetic blueprint.

- **Mixtures and Mingle Mystery:** Dive into the mixtures and mingle mystery, where the coexistence of multiple DNA sources poses a forensic conundrum. Probability equations and statistical models become tools to untangle the intricacies.

- **Phenomenal PCR Artistry:** Witness the phenomenal PCR artistry addressing minute DNA quantities. In the realm of low-copy-number DNA, the delicate dance of polymerase chain reaction (PCR) amplification becomes a forensic masterpiece.

- **Interpreting Complex Profiles Ballet:** Engage in the interpreting complex profiles ballet, where complex DNA profiles challenge forensic analysts. Statistical algorithms perform a choreography of interpretation, distinguishing signal from noise.

- **Striking a Balance Equation:** Picture the delicate balance equation between sensitivity and specificity in DNA analysis. Striving for a method that captures faint traces without compromising accuracy is the forensic scientist's equilibrium act.

- **Technological Evolution Symphony:** Experience the technological evolution symphony, as innovations in next-generation sequencing and advanced analytical tools reshape the landscape of DNA analysis, opening new frontiers and presenting novel challenges.

- **Ethical Dilemmas Sonata:** Delve into the ethical dilemmas sonata, where the power of DNA raises questions of privacy, consent, and the responsible use of genetic information, prompting a harmonious balance between justice and individual rights.

In the intricate dance of DNA analysis challenges, forensic science advances, weaving a narrative of perseverance, innovation, and the relentless pursuit of truth.

18.8   Cold Cases and DNA

Unlock the mysteries of unresolved cases as DNA takes center stage:

- **DNA Time Capsules:** Envision DNA as a time-traveling detective. In cold cases, preserved DNA becomes a silent witness, waiting for the right technology to unveil its secrets.

- **Advancements in DNA Technologies:** Imagine the leap from the past to the present. Modern DNA analysis techniques, like STR profiling and mitochondrial DNA sequencing, breathe life into dormant cases.

- **Genetic Genealogy Revolution:** Picture a genealogical map guiding investigations. Genetic genealogy, powered by DNA databases, redefines family trees, unearthing connections and solving long-standing mysteries.

- **Familial DNA Searching:** Navigate the ethical landscape of familial DNA searching. Uncover leads by identifying relatives, bringing investigators closer to solving cases.

- **Isotopic Analysis:** Visualize isotopes revealing geographical secrets. This multidisciplinary approach, combined with DNA analysis, provides a holistic view, reconstructing the stories of unidentified victims.

In the realm of cold cases, DNA emerges as the key, transcending time to deliver justice.

Chapter 19

Forensic Psychiatry

19.1 Introduction to Forensic Psychiatry

Delve into the intersection of law and mental health:

- **Psychiatry meets Legal System:** Imagine the courtroom as a stage for the mind. Forensic psychiatry merges psychiatric expertise with legal matters, assessing mental states in legal contexts.

- **Insanity Defense Formula:** Encounter the legal formula for insanity. Insanity is often defined as a mental disorder preventing one from understanding the consequences of their actions or distinguishing right from wrong.

- **Competency to Stand Trial:** Decode the mental fitness criteria. Evaluations determine if an individual is competent to participate in legal proceedings, understanding charges and assisting in their defense.

- **Risk Assessment Models:** Navigate the complexities of risk evaluation. Forensic psychiatrists use models to predict future behaviors, aiding in parole decisions and community safety.

- **Psychopathy and Criminality:** Uncover the psyche of criminals. Psychopathy, a personality disorder, is often linked to criminal behavior, influencing legal decisions and sentencing.

In the realm of Forensic Psychiatry, the intricacies of the mind intertwine with the demands of the legal system.

19.2   Criminal Responsibility

Unravel the web of responsibility in the realm of crime and mental health:

- **M'Naghten Rule:** Enter the arena of legal sanity. The M'Naghten Rule sets the standard for criminal responsibility, focusing on the accused's ability to distinguish right from wrong at the time of the crime.

- **Irresistible Impulse Test:** Explore the concept of impulse control. This test examines whether a defendant, due to mental illness, could control their actions, even if they knew the actions were wrong.

- **Durham Rule:** Witness the evolution of legal standards. The Durham Rule considers whether the accused's unlawful act was a product of their mental disorder, expanding the scope of insanity defenses.

- **ALI Test:** Confront the complexities of legal insanity. The American Law Institute (ALI) Test combines cognitive and volitional elements, evaluating if the defendant, due to mental disorder, lacked substantial capacity to conform their conduct to the law.

- **Diminished Capacity:** Navigate the nuances of partial responsibility. Some jurisdictions recognize diminished capacity as a mitigating factor, acknowledging mental conditions that fall short of legal insanity.

In the landscape of Criminal Responsibility, the interplay between the mind's intricacies and legal culpability takes center stage.

19.3   Competency to Stand Trial

Enter the courtroom where mental fitness meets legal proceedings:

- **Dusky Standard:** Gauge the defendant's courtroom readiness. The Dusky Standard demands that the accused must possess a rational and factual understanding of the proceedings and be able to assist their attorney.

- **Competency Evaluation:** Witness the psychiatric scrutiny. Competency evaluations, conducted by mental health professionals, delve into the defendant's mental state, ensuring they can comprehend the charges and participate in their defense.

- **Restoration to Competency:** Navigate the path to trial readiness. If found incompetent, defendants undergo treatment to restore competency, bridging the gap between mental health and legal proceedings.

- **Legal vs. Clinical Competency:** Uncover the dual nature of competency. While clinical competency focuses on mental well-being, legal competency emphasizes the ability to engage in the legal process, striking a balance between mental health and judicial efficacy.

- **Interdisciplinary Collaboration:** Explore the synergy between law and psychiatry. Competency assessments often involve collaboration between legal and mental health professionals, combining expertise to ensure a fair trial.

In the realm of Competency to Stand Trial, the intersection of mental capacity and legal fitness takes precedence.

19.4   Insanity Defense

Step into the courtroom where sanity meets culpability:

- **M'Naghten Rule:** Unravel the criteria for insanity. The M'Naghten Rule scrutinizes whether the accused, due to mental illness, knew the nature of their actions or understood that they were wrong.

- **Irresistible Impulse Test:** Probe the impulse of mental illness. This test explores whether the defendant, even if knowing the act was wrong, was unable to control their actions due to an irresistible impulse.

- **Durham Rule:** Witness the expansion of insanity considerations. The Durham Rule broadens the scope, attributing criminal acts to a mental disease or defect, encompassing a wider range of psychiatric conditions.

- **Insanity Reform:** Navigate the evolution of insanity defense. Jurisdictions may adopt variations of insanity standards, reflecting societal perceptions and advancements in psychiatric understanding.

- **Diminished Capacity:** Delve into nuances of culpability. Some jurisdictions consider diminished capacity as a mitigating factor, reducing the degree of responsibility based on the defendant's mental state.

In the arena of the Insanity Defense, the delicate balance between mental health and legal culpability takes center stage.

19.5 Psychological Autopsy

Unlocking the secrets of the mind after death:

- **Post-Mortem Profiling:** Imagine a detective probing the psyche. Psychological autopsy reconstructs the mental state of the deceased, analyzing medical records, interviews, and contextual information.

- **Suicide Investigations:** Navigate the complexities of self-inflicted death. Psychological autopsy aids in understanding motives, mental health factors, and circumstances surrounding suicides, assisting in investigations.

- **Profiling Mental States:** Picture deciphering the clues left in behavior. Psychiatric professionals unravel the psychological puzzle, shedding light on mental illnesses, stressors, or external factors influencing the individual.

- **Forensic Psychiatry Expertise:** Envision mental health experts collaborating with investigators. Their insights contribute to a comprehensive understanding of the deceased's mental well-being, offering a unique perspective in legal contexts.

- **Preventing Future Tragedies:** Consider the potential for prevention. Insights gained from psychological autopsies contribute to mental health awareness, intervention strategies, and, ultimately, the prevention of similar incidents.

In the realm of the Psychological Autopsy, the post-mortem exploration of the mind adds a nuanced layer to forensic investigations.

19.6 Risk Assessment

Deciphering the potential for future harm:

- **Predictive Profiling:** Imagine foreseeing potential threats. Risk assessment in forensic psychiatry involves evaluating factors that may indicate future violent behavior, aiding in preventive measures.

- **Clinical Formulas:** Picture a formula for danger. Psychiatric professionals employ structured risk assessment tools, combining clinical expertise and statistical models to quantify and predict the risk of harm.

- **Dynamic Factors:** Envision a constantly evolving analysis. Risk assessment considers dynamic factors, such as changes in mental health, substance use, or life circumstances, ensuring ongoing accuracy.

- **Preventive Interventions:** Picture interventions before harm occurs. Assessing risk allows for tailored interventions, including therapy, monitoring, or institutionalization, to mitigate potential dangers.

- **Legal Implications:** Consider the intersection of psychiatry and law. Risk assessments influence legal decisions, informing judgments related to involuntary commitments, parole, and other legal proceedings.

In the realm of Risk Assessment, forensic psychiatry becomes a proactive force in safeguarding individuals and communities.

19.7   Mental Health Laws

Navigating the legal landscape of mental health:

- **Involuntary Commitment Formula:** Envision a balance between autonomy and safety. Mental health laws provide a formula for involuntary commitment, weighing the individual's rights against the need for protection.

- **Capacity Equations:** Picture a legal measure of mental capacity. Laws define formulas to assess a person's mental capacity, influencing decisions on consent, guardianship, and the ability to stand trial.

- **Legal Insanity Criteria:** Imagine a standardized test for legal insanity. Mental health laws establish criteria, often involving cognitive impairment or inability to understand the consequences of actions, to determine legal insanity.

- **Civil vs. Criminal Formulas:** Consider the dichotomy of civil and criminal aspects. Mental health laws distinguish formulas for civil commitment, focused on treatment, and criminal commitment, addressing legal consequences for offenses.

- **Ethical Considerations:** Reflect on the ethical dimensions. Mental health laws incorporate ethical principles, ensuring a balance between individual rights, public safety, and the principles of beneficence and non-maleficence.

In the complex realm of Mental Health Laws, the legal system intertwines with psychiatric principles to navigate issues of personal freedom, treatment, and societal protection.

19.8   Psychological Profiling

Unlocking the mysteries of the mind in forensic investigations:

- **Criminal Mind Equations:** Imagine decoding criminal behavior. Psychological profiling involves creating equations that analyze crime scenes, victimology, and offender behavior to unveil patterns and motives.

- **Personality Formulas:** Envision the science of personality unraveling crimes. Profilers use established formulas to assess personality traits, helping create a psychological profile that aids in suspect identification.

- **Geographical Analysis:** Picture mapping the criminal mind. Profilers integrate geographic equations to understand how offenders select and navigate crime scenes, providing insights into their mental processes.

- **Serial Offender Algorithms:** Consider algorithms identifying serial patterns. Profiling utilizes mathematical models to recognize patterns across multiple crimes, aiding law enforcement in connecting seemingly unrelated cases.

- **Behavioral Equations:** Reflect on the equation of behavior. Profilers develop formulas to interpret behavioral cues, helping law enforcement anticipate an offender's next moves and devise effective investigative strategies.

In the realm of Psychological Profiling, equations and algorithms become tools to unravel the intricate threads of criminal behavior and aid investigators in solving complex cases.

Chapter 20

Forensic Ballistics

20.1   Introduction to Forensic Ballistics

Unveiling the secrets of projectiles and firearms in forensic investigations:

- **Bullet Trajectory Formula:** Imagine tracing the path of justice. Forensic ballistics employs trajectory formulas, considering factors like gravity and air resistance, to pinpoint the exact path a bullet travels.

- **Firearm Identification Equation:** Envision linking a bullet to its source. Unique markings on bullets and cartridge cases are decoded using mathematical equations, establishing a firearm's identity.

- **Gunshot Residue Analysis:** Picture unraveling the aftermath of a shot. Formulas in gunshot residue analysis detect particles, confirming if a suspect fired a weapon recently.

- **Firearm Mechanisms Formula:** Consider the mechanics behind the trigger. Forensic ballistics involves understanding firearm mechanisms through equations, shedding light on how guns operate.

- **Virtual Reconstruction Algorithm:** Visualize reconstructing a crime in the virtual realm. Forensic ballistics employs algorithms to recreate shooting incidents, aiding in crime scene analysis.

In the domain of Forensic Ballistics, formulas and equations become the ammunition that investigators deploy to piece together the narratives hidden within bullets and firearms.

20.2　Firearm Types and Mechanisms

Unlock the mysteries of firearms with a glimpse into their diverse types and intricate mechanisms:

- **Bullet Kinetic Energy Formula:** Imagine the energy behind a bullet. The kinetic energy formula calculates the energy possessed by a bullet, offering insights into its potential impact.

- **Firearm Action Equations:** Envision the dynamics of firearm actions. Different equations reveal the mechanics of bolt-action, semi-automatic, and automatic firearms, unraveling their distinct operating systems.

- **Recoil Force Calculation:** Picture the backward force of a shot. Formulas for recoil force consider bullet mass, velocity, and firearm weight, providing a quantitative measure of the kick a shooter experiences.

- **Chamber Pressure Analysis:** Visualize the pressure within a firearm. Equations assessing chamber pressure help understand the internal forces during firing, crucial for both forensic analysis and firearm design.

- **Gunpowder Burn Rate Experiment:** Consider the burn rate of gunpowder. Experimental setups and chemical equations explore how different gunpowder compositions burn, influencing bullet propulsion.

In the realm of Forensic Ballistics, formulas and equations unravel the secrets held within firearms, shedding light on their characteristics and behaviors.

20.3　Bullet and Cartridge Case Examination

Dive into the world of bullets and cartridge cases, unlocking their stories through examination:

- **Bullet Striation Analysis:** Imagine bullet markings as unique signatures. Striation analysis involves comparing the microscopic marks on bullets, aiding in firearm identification.

- **Bullet Caliber Measurement Formula:** Picture determining bullet caliber. The formula, involving measurements of the bullet's diameter, assists in narrowing down the type of firearm used.

- **Cartridge Case Headstamp Decoding:** Visualize decoding cartridge cases. Understanding headstamp markings on cases reveals valuable information about the ammunition manufacturer and production batch.

- **Firearm Identification Equations:** Envision matching bullets and cases to specific firearms. Identification equations consider factors like rifling characteristics, firing pin impressions, and ejector marks.

- **Gunshot Residue (GSR) Chemical Test:** Explore GSR analysis. Chemical equations unveil the presence of gunshot residue elements, crucial in determining a shooter's proximity to a discharged firearm.

In the realm of Forensic Ballistics, formulas and examinations transform bullets and cartridge cases into forensic storytellers, aiding investigators in solving mysteries.

20.4 Bullet Trajectory Analysis

Embark on a journey tracing the path of bullets with the precision of trajectory analysis:

- **Trajectory Calculation Formula:** Envision calculating bullet paths. The trajectory formula factors in the initial velocity, angle of projection, and gravitational pull, unraveling the journey of a projectile.

- **Use of Laser Technology:** Picture lasers mapping bullet trajectories. Advanced technology, combined with mathematical calculations, assists in reconstructing the precise path a bullet takes through space.

- **Impact Angle Determination:** Visualize determining the angle of impact. Formulas involving the entry and exit points of a projectile help establish the angle, crucial for understanding the dynamics of a shooting incident.

- **Bloodstain Pattern Analysis:** Explore the intersection of ballistics and bloodstains. Understanding the interaction between bullets and blood aids investigators in reconstructing the sequence of events.

- **3D Crime Scene Mapping:** Envision crime scenes in three dimensions. Modern techniques incorporate trajectory analysis into 3D mapping, providing a comprehensive view of how bullets traverse space.

In the domain of Forensic Ballistics, bullet trajectories become mathematical narratives, unraveling the mysteries of shooting incidents.

20.5 Gunshot Residue Analysis

Dive into the microscopic world of gunshot residue (GSR) with a glimpse of formulas and analysis techniques:

- **Composition of GSR:** Imagine the elements unveiling the shooter. GSR primarily consists of lead, barium, and antimony. Detecting and quantifying these elements offer crucial insights.

- **Distance Estimation Formula:** Visualize calculating the shooting distance. The GSR distribution on a target follows a mathematical relationship, aiding investigators in approximating how far the shot was fired.

- **Scanning Electron Microscopy (SEM):** Picture microscopic examination. SEM allows detailed visualization of GSR particles, enabling forensic experts to analyze their morphology and composition.

- **X-ray Spectroscopy:** Envision elemental analysis with X-rays. Techniques like Energy Dispersive X-ray Spectroscopy (EDX) help identify and quantify the specific elements present in GSR.

- **Molecular Analysis:** Explore the molecular fingerprints. Advanced methods delve into organic compounds associated with firearms, adding a molecular layer to GSR analysis.

In the realm of Gunshot Residue Analysis, elements and formulas converge to tell the story of a discharged firearm.

20.6 Firearm Identification

Unveil the secrets hidden in the barrels and breeches as we explore firearm identification with a touch of formulas and forensic chemistry:

- **Striations and Rifling:** Imagine the uniqueness of barrel patterns. Firearm examiners analyze striations and rifling marks left on bullets, turning the barrel's twists into distinct fingerprints.

- **Caliber Determination Formula:** Visualize deducing the caliber from a bullet. The relationship between bullet diameter, lands, and grooves provides a formulaic approach to narrowing down the firearm type.

- **Bullet Casing Analysis:** Picture the chemistry of firing. Chemical signatures from primer compounds, propellants, and gunshot residue on casings contribute to identifying the type of ammunition and, potentially, the firearm.

- **Toolmark Analysis:** Envision matching the tools to the crime. Toolmarks left on cartridges and bullets, resulting from manufacturing processes, become integral in linking firearms to specific tools.

- **Chemical Signature of Gunpowder:** Explore the molecular realm. Identifying specific chemical compounds in gunpowder residues adds a chemical fingerprint to the investigation.

In the realm of Firearm Identification, formulas and chemical signatures create a symphony, harmonizing the language of ballistics.

20.7   Toolmarks in Ballistics

Unraveling mysteries etched in metal surfaces, the world of Toolmarks in Ballistics comes alive with a blend of formulas and chemical insights:

- **Striagraphy Principles:** Imagine reading tool stories. Striagraphy, akin to geography for tools, decodes the topography of toolmarks, revealing the unique landscape of their surfaces.

- **Toolmark Impressions:** Visualize the artistry of tool interaction. Toolmark impressions on bullets and casings become distinctive signatures, providing clues to the tools' characteristics.

- **IBIS Technology:** Enter the realm of cutting-edge ballistics. Integrated Ballistic Identification Systems (IBIS) use advanced imaging and comparison algorithms to match toolmarks, enhancing investigative efficiency.

- **Chemical Analysis of Toolmarks:** Peer into the molecular canvas. Chemical analysis of toolmarks involves detecting trace elements, providing additional layers of evidence through the unique elemental signatures of tools.

- **Fractography:** Envision the fractures telling tales. Fractography studies the patterns of fractures on surfaces, aiding in understanding the dynamics of tool interactions and helping link tools to specific incidents.

In Toolmarks in Ballistics, formulas and chemical nuances bring the language of tools to life, creating a symphony of clues for forensic investigators.

20.8   Virtual Reconstruction in Ballistics

Embark on a digital journey where bullets and trajectories find new life through Virtual Reconstruction in Ballistics. Fast-track your understanding with a fusion of formulas and digital magic:

- **3D Trajectory Modeling:** Picture the flight path. Utilizing 3D trajectory models, investigators simulate bullet paths, reconstructing the dynamics of shooting incidents with mathematical precision.

- **Physics of Ballistic Trajectories:** Dive into the formulas behind motion. Equations of motion and projectile dynamics unravel the physics of ballistic trajectories, transforming crime scenes into mathematical puzzles.

- **Digital Crime Scene Mapping:** Visualize crime scenes in bits and bytes. Virtual Reconstruction employs digital mapping tools to recreate crime scenes, offering a panoramic view that aids in trajectory analysis.

- **Forensic Animation:** Bring bullet trajectories to life. Forensic animation techniques transform static data into dynamic visualizations, enhancing the courtroom experience and making complex ballistics concepts accessible.

- **Virtual Reality (VR) Simulations:** Step into the virtual crime scene. VR simulations allow investigators to explore shooting incidents firsthand, providing a unique perspective for analysis and courtroom presentations.

In Virtual Reconstruction in Ballistics, the fusion of formulas and digital innovation opens a new chapter in forensic investigations, where the virtual realm becomes a powerful ally.

Chapter 21

Digital Forensics

21.1   Introduction to Digital Forensics

Unveil the digital realm where every byte tells a story. In the world of Digital Forensics, speed meets complexity, and formulas unveil secrets:

- **Digital Evidence Triad:** Imagine the trinity of data – storage, processing, and communication. Digital forensics explores the interplay, dissecting devices to extract evidence from hard drives, volatile memory, and communication channels.

- **Hash Functions:** Dive into the world of hash values. Mathematical magic ensures data integrity with hash functions, allowing investigators to verify the authenticity of digital evidence.

- **Timeline Analysis:** Picture timelines narrating digital sagas. Creating chronological sequences of events, timeline analysis reconstructs the digital journey, uncovering the who, what, and when of cyber incidents.

- **File Carving:** Envision data resurrection. File carving algorithms sift through digital remnants, extracting files from fragmented or damaged storage media, piecing together the puzzle of deleted or corrupted data.

- **Network Forensics Equations:** Decode the language of networks. Equations in network forensics reveal patterns, anomalies, and traces of cyber activities, transforming raw data into actionable intelligence.

In the symphony of zeros and ones, Digital Forensics emerges as the maestro, conducting investigations in the ever-expanding landscape of digital evidence.

21.2   Computer and Mobile Device Analysis

Embark on the journey of unraveling digital mysteries within computers and mobile devices. In this realm, where bits and bytes hold the keys, let's explore the essentials:

- **Forensic Imaging:** Picture creating a digital clone. Forensic imaging captures every nook and cranny of storage media, preserving an exact replica for investigation without altering the original.

- **File System Analysis:** Delve into the structure of digital organization. File systems hold the blueprint, and their analysis unveils the hierarchy, metadata, and relationships, exposing the narrative of digital activities.

- **Mobile Forensics Formulas:** Imagine decoding the language of smartphones. Formulas in mobile forensics dissect mobile operating systems, extracting call logs, messages, and app data, constructing a timeline of user interactions.

- **Cloud Forensics Equations:** Navigate the cloud's ethereal landscape. Equations in cloud forensics decipher virtual trails, accessing data stored across remote servers, bringing transparency to cloud-based activities.

- **Recovery Techniques:** Envision data resurrection. Recovery techniques breathe life into deleted files. Whether it's a wiped hard drive or a formatted memory card, these techniques recover digital echoes, crucial for investigations.

In the world of Computer and Mobile Device Analysis, each equation unveils a piece of the digital puzzle, aiding investigators in reconstructing the narrative of cyber incidents.

21.3   File Systems and Data Recovery

Embark on a digital quest into the heart of file systems and the art of data resurrection. Let's unravel this section with speed and clarity:

- **File System Dynamics:** Imagine file systems as the architects of digital landscapes. Understanding their dynamics, equations unveil the intricate structures, attributes, and relationships within, guiding investigators through the data terrain.

- **Deleted Data Alchemy:** Picture deleted data as hidden treasure. Forensic formulas perform alchemy, resurrecting seemingly lost files. Through intricate algorithms, investigators breathe life into the remnants of digital existence.

- **Data Recovery Molecular Equation:** Envision data recovery as a molecular process. With precision and finesse, the molecular equation orchestrates the revival of bits and bytes, reconstructing the fabric of digital information.

- **Entropy of Erasure:** Navigate the entropy of erasure. This formula quantifies the degree of data obliteration, crucial for assessing intentional data destruction or uncovering traces left by sophisticated digital adversaries.

- **Temporal Redundancy Formula:** Uncover the temporal redundancy in data. Like a forensic clock, this formula helps reconstruct timelines by identifying remnants of past data states, aiding investigators in piecing together the chronology of digital events.

In the realm of File Systems and Data Recovery, these formulas illuminate the path from digital obscurity to clarity, empowering investigators to resurrect and decipher the hidden narratives within digital realms.

21.4 Network Forensics

Dive into the labyrinth of cyberspace and unravel the secrets of Network Forensics. Fast-track through this section with formulas that illuminate the digital trails:

- **Packet Sniffing Formula:** Envision the digital senses at work. Packet sniffing formula, the olfactory system of network forensics, captures and analyzes data packets, unveiling hidden scents of cyber activity.

- **Network Traffic Entropy:** Picture the chaos and order within network traffic. The entropy formula quantifies the randomness or predictability, aiding investigators in identifying anomalies that may signify malicious activities.

- **Cyber Time Travel Equation:** Time travel in cyberspace? Almost. This equation reconstructs the sequence of cyber events, acting as a temporal compass for investigators navigating through the digital chronicles.

- **Forensic Hash Function:** Imagine a digital fingerprint for every file. The forensic hash function formula generates unique identifiers, enabling investigators to verify data integrity and identify alterations in the digital landscape.

- **Malware Propagation Reaction:** Witness the spread of digital infections. Modeled like a chemical reaction, this formula illustrates the dynamics of malware propagation through networks, aiding in containment and eradication strategies.

In the realm of Network Forensics, these formulas serve as beacons, guiding investigators through the intricate web of cyber incidents, where every equation unveils a layer of the digital mystery.

21.5 Cybercrime Investigations

Embark on a digital pursuit as Cybercrime Investigations unfold, illuminated by formulas that cut through the virtual fog:

- **Digital Evidence Accumulation:** Picture the data reservoir. The formula for digital evidence accumulation quantifies the relevance and weight of electronic artifacts, constructing a foundation for legal proceedings.

- **Forensic Triangulation Equation:** Navigate the maze of digital footprints. The forensic triangulation equation integrates multiple sources of digital evidence, converging on the truth and eliminating false leads.

- **Incident Severity Index:** Gauge the impact of cyber incidents. The incident severity index formula assigns a numerical value, allowing investigators to prioritize responses based on the potential harm to digital assets.

- **Cryptographic Puzzle Solver:** Decrypt the enigma of encrypted data. The cryptographic puzzle solver formula, akin to a chemical reaction, unravels coded messages, exposing hidden motives and plans.

- **Digital Alibi Verification:** Uncover the alibis in the digital realm. This formula cross-references timelines, verifying or disproving digital alibis, crucial in establishing or debunking suspect narratives.

In the world of Cybercrime Investigations, these formulas act as digital torchbearers, illuminating the path to truth and justice amidst the complexities of the virtual landscape.

21.6 Forensic Analysis of Malware

Delve into the realm of malicious code and digital detectives with formulas illuminating the analysis process:

- **Malware Signature Matching:** Envision a digital fingerprint. The formula for malware signature matching compares binary patterns, unveiling the identity of malicious code and its variants.

- **Code Entropy Calculation:** Peer into the chaos of code. The code entropy calculation formula quantifies the randomness within a program, aiding in distinguishing normal code from obfuscated or malicious ones.

- **Propagation Rate Equation:** Witness the digital contagion. The propagation rate equation models the speed at which malware spreads, aiding in containment strategies and understanding the scope of an outbreak.

- **Decryption Key Recovery:** Crack the code's secret language. The decryption key recovery formula, akin to solving a chemical equation, retrieves keys from encrypted malware, enabling the restoration of compromised data.

- **Forensic Hash Analysis:** Picture a digital fingerprint database. The forensic hash analysis formula cross-references hashes, identifying known malware specimens and streamlining the investigation process.

In the field of Forensic Analysis of Malware, these formulas serve as the digital microscope, unraveling the intricacies of malicious digital landscapes.

21.7   Digital Evidence Handling

Navigate the intricate terrain of digital evidence with these streamlined formulas:

- **Chain of Custody Formula:** Imagine a secure digital handoff. The chain of custody formula ensures the integrity of digital evidence, detailing every custodian change to maintain admissibility.

- **Forensic Imaging Efficiency:** Picture a digital Xerox machine. The forensic imaging efficiency formula gauges the speed of creating a bit-for-bit copy, preserving evidence without altering the original.

- **Data Recovery Success Rate:** Gauge the chances of resurrection. The data recovery success rate formula predicts the probability of extracting relevant information from damaged or deleted digital artifacts.

- **Entropy in File Analysis:** Peer into the randomness of files. The entropy in file analysis formula quantifies disorder, aiding in identifying encrypted or compressed files within the digital haystack.

- **Metadata Reconstruction:** Reconstruct the digital crime scene. The metadata reconstruction formula helps rebuild the context by piecing together digital breadcrumbs, such as timestamps and file attributes.

In the realm of Digital Evidence Handling, these formulas act as digital Swiss army knives, ensuring the precision and reliability of digital forensic investigations.

21.8   Legal Issues in Digital Forensics

Decode the legal landscape of digital forensics with these concise formulas:

- **Legal Admissibility Formula:** Envision a digital evidence passport. The legal admissibility formula verifies the authenticity and integrity of digital evidence, ensuring its acceptance in court.

- **Authentication Confidence:** Gauge the trustworthiness of digital fingerprints. The authentication confidence formula assesses the reliability of digital evidence, critical for establishing its probative value.

- **Expert Witness Credibility:** Picture the forensic virtuoso on the stand. The expert witness credibility formula combines expertise, communication, and demeanor to enhance the persuasiveness of digital forensic testimony.

- **Legal Challenges Resilience:** Navigate the courtroom battlefield. The legal challenges resilience formula prepares digital forensic experts for potential legal challenges, fortifying their methodologies and findings.

- **Privacy Preservation Equation:** Safeguard digital rights. The privacy preservation equation balances the investigative need with individual privacy, ensuring a lawful and ethical approach to digital evidence collection.

In the realm of Legal Issues in Digital Forensics, these formulas serve as legal compasses, guiding digital investigators through the intricate terrain of the legal system.

Chapter 22

Conclusion

22.1 Summary of Key Findings

Summarize the investigative journey with these memorable highlights:

- **Forensic Equation of Discovery:** Imagine the investigative formula unveiling hidden truths. The forensic equation of discovery integrates evidence, analysis, and deduction to unravel mysteries.

- **Information Entropy Principle:** Picture the digital universe's unraveling. The information entropy principle quantifies the degree of surprise in findings, emphasizing the significance of unexpected discoveries in forensic investigations.

- **Probabilistic Certainty Theorem:** Gauge the strength of investigative conclusions. The probabilistic certainty theorem balances probabilities, providing a nuanced understanding of the certainty associated with forensic findings.

- **Ethical Inquiry Constant:** Navigate the ethical dimensions of investigation. The ethical inquiry constant ensures that investigative practices align with ethical standards, fostering trust in forensic processes.

- **Justice Optimization Algorithm:** Envision justice as an algorithm. The justice optimization algorithm strives to maximize fairness, accuracy, and integrity in forensic outcomes, emphasizing the ultimate goal of serving justice.

In conclusion, these formulas encapsulate the essence of forensic investigations, where science, technology, and ethics converge to illuminate the truth.

22.2 Contributions to Forensic Medicine

Celebrate the profound impact on forensic medicine with these key contributions:

- **Forensic Advancement Quotient (FAQ):** Measure the progress in forensic medicine. The FAQ combines technological advancements, research breakthroughs, and improved methodologies, reflecting the dynamic evolution of forensic practices.

- **Mortality Clarity Index (MCI):** Illuminate the understanding of mortality patterns. The MCI dissects mortality data, revealing patterns and trends that contribute to a comprehensive grasp of forensic medicine's role in understanding and preventing fatalities.

- **Pathological Resilience Coefficient (PRC):** Assess the resilience of forensic methodologies. The PRC gauges the robustness of forensic techniques in the face of challenges, ensuring adaptability and effectiveness in diverse investigative scenarios.

- **Toxicological Harmony Constant (THC):** Achieve balance in toxicological investigations. The THC symbolizes the equilibrium between substance analysis and interpretation, harmonizing toxicological findings for accurate forensic assessments.

- **Genomic Justice Quotient (GJQ):** Embrace the genomic era in forensic medicine. The GJQ quantifies the integration of genomic insights, ensuring that forensic practices align with cutting-edge genetic advancements for precise identification and analysis.

In summary, these formulas encapsulate the enduring contributions of forensic medicine, where innovation, resilience, and precision converge to enhance our understanding of mortality and contribute to the pursuit of justice.

22.3 Challenges and Future Directions

Navigate the challenges and chart the future course of forensic endeavors with these insightful formulations:

- **Obstacle Overcoming Coefficient (OOC):** Quantify the ability to overcome challenges. The OOC assesses the forensic field's resilience, measuring how effectively it tackles obstacles, adapts to evolving scenarios, and maintains investigative momentum.

- **Innovation Integration Index (III):** Gauge the integration of innovation. The III evaluates how seamlessly forensic practices incorporate technological advancements, research breakthroughs, and novel methodologies, ensuring a forward-looking and dynamic approach.

- **Collaboration Catalyst Quotient (CCQ):** Measure the impact of collaboration. The CCQ assesses the strength of interdisciplinary collaborations, fostering a symbiotic relationship between forensic medicine, law enforcement, and other relevant fields to enhance investigative capacities.

- **Technological Trajectory Rate (TTR):** Predict the trajectory of technology. The TTR extrapolates the pace at which technology is likely to evolve within the forensic landscape, providing foresight for research and resource allocation in anticipation of future technological advancements.

- **Global Forensic Footprint (GFF):** Evaluate the global impact of forensic efforts. The GFF calculates the reach and influence of forensic practices on a global scale, emphasizing the importance of international collaboration and the dissemination of forensic knowledge.

In addressing challenges and setting future directions, these formulas serve as beacons, guiding the forensic community toward innovative solutions, collaborative ventures, and a technologically enriched landscape.

22.4 Closing Remarks

Concluding our forensic journey with impactful insights and resonant formulas:

- **Justice Dispensation Quotient (JDQ):** Reflect on the efficiency of forensic contributions. The JDQ encapsulates the effectiveness of forensic practices in ensuring justice, considering the speed, accuracy, and fairness with which investigations lead to legal outcomes.

- **Truth Unveiling Index (TUI):** Gauge the commitment to uncovering truth. The TUI measures the dedication of forensic professionals to unveil the facts, emphasizing the pursuit of truth as the ultimate goal in every investigation.

- **Ethical Equilibrium Constant (EEC):** Ensure ethical standards in forensic endeavors. The EEC evaluates the balance between scientific advancements and ethical considerations, promoting a harmonious integration that upholds moral values and safeguards the integrity of forensic processes.

- **Humanitarian Impact Factor (HIF):** Assess the impact on individuals and society. The HIF quantifies the positive influence of forensic work on human lives, emphasizing the humanitarian aspects and societal benefits derived from advancements in forensic medicine.

- **Legacy Continuation Coefficient (LCC):** Consider the lasting legacy of forensic contributions. The LCC measures the sustainability and enduring impact of forensic practices, ensuring that advancements made today continue to shape the future landscape of forensic medicine.

As we bid farewell to this exploration, may these formulas resonate, underscoring the ongoing commitment to truth, justice, and ethical principles in the realm of forensic sciences.